The Green Pregnancy Diet

Healthy eating habits for mommy, baby, and the planet

Radha McLean

Nutrition editor: Tara Gidus, RD
Contributing author: Thauna Abrin, ND

iUniverse, Inc.
New York   Bloomington

The Green Pregnancy Diet
Healthy eating habits for mommy, baby, and the planet

You should not undertake any diet/exercise regimen recommended in this book before consulting your personal physician. Neither the author nor the publisher shall be responsible or liable for any loss or damage allegedly arising as a consequence of your use or application of any information or suggestions contained in this book.
iUniverse books may be ordered through booksellers or by contacting:

iUniverse
1663 Liberty Drive
Bloomington, IN 47403
www.iuniverse.com
1-800-Authors (1-800-288-4677)

Because of the dynamic nature of the Internet, any Web addresses or links contained in this book may have changed since publication and may no longer be valid. The views expressed in this work are solely those of the author and do not necessarily reflect the views of the publisher, and the publisher hereby disclaims any responsibility for them.

ISBN: 978-1-4401-1229-4 (pbk)
ISBN: 978-1-4401-1230-0 (ebk)

Printed in the United States of America

iUniverse rev. date: 3/25/09

Contents

Breakfast

Snacks

Lunch & Dinner

Desserts

Introduction

Pregnancy is an exciting time meant to be enjoyed and celebrated with family and friends. You have one problem, however: You're constantly hungry! You want to eat everything in sight, but have your health and that of your unborn baby to think of before inhaling that extra slice of pizza and can of diet soda. "What should I eat *now*?" you may be asking yourself at every meal and at snack times.

The quality of the food you eat is continually on your mind, and the gamut of health issues you now need to consider can make your head spin. First, you want to eat nutritious food. Then, you need to keep an eye out for the mercury in fish, and the chemicals and additives in conventional meats, dairy products, fruits, and vegetables. To complicate matters, you should try to avoid toxins lurking in the kitchen, which can be found in everything from tap water and cleaning supplies to pans and plastic containers used to store food.

Here's the good news: eating a nutritious, nontoxic, and environmentally-friendly diet during your pregnancy is easier than you think. Take as a case in point the transformation I made when I got pregnant.

As a lifelong lacto-vegetarian who does not eat eggs or fish (my mother became a vegetarian before I was conceived), I ate whole and refined grains, beans, dairy, vegetables, fruits, and desserts. But my diet had a few essential flaws—flaws far too common in the eating habits of many women today. I often ate "on the run," overlooking the nutrients and chemical additives in my meals. Plus, I treated myself to snacks made of refined carbohydrates, or "empty carbs"—foods high in sugar and low in nutrients like ice cream and cookies—to curb my cravings for sweets.

Everything changed when I got pregnant. My first trimester was plagued with uncontrollable hunger. I was starving all the time! I needed to start eating nutritious food more consistently—for every meal and snack, which would fill me up for longer periods of time. Also, even though I was taking a prenatal vitamin, I had no idea if I was getting enough of the major nutrients important for the health of my unborn baby, such as iron, protein and omega-3 fats. In addition, I felt panicked about the toxic chemicals and additives found in so many packaged and conventionally grown (nonorganic) foods. These chemicals could harm the health of my baby! Plus, I wanted to start eating a diet that was more environmentally-friendly. Now that I was bringing a child (a boy) into the world, I wanted to help keep it a safe place for him to live.

How could I address all of these concerns?

Simple. I needed to change my diet. I did research on my own and consulted with a number of healthcare experts, including contributing author Thauna Abrin, ND, a naturopathic doctor and trained midwife who is also my sister. I adapted the meal recommendations I received to meet my lifestyle requirement—most with preparation time of fifteen minutes or less. The result was a healthy diet of meals that

- Were easy to make
- Included nutrients important to get during pregnancy
- Used whole grain, nontoxic, environmentally-friendly ingredients
- Curbed my food cravings
- Tasted good!

Next, I made a few, basic changes to my kitchen supplies and habits to keep environmental toxins out of my kitchen and cut down on waste. Before I knew it, I was eating green and feeling great.

The information I used to make my transformation is found in this book:

- Basic tips on how to eat a nontoxic, environmentally-friendly diet
- Simple definitions of the different nutrients, food groups and portion sizes you need during your pregnancy
- Explanations of the toxins in kitchen products that could be harmful, and easy ways to avoid them
- Tips on ways to have an environmentally-friendly kitchen
- Quick, nutritious, and flavorful recipes without the added toxins, chemicals or empty carbs
  With the wealth of green lifestyle and healthy food choices now available, it has never been easier to start eating green during your pregnancy—when it counts most.

The information in this book is not intended as medical advice; it's more of a guide to help you make greener eating choices. Consult with your healthcare provider if you have questions about pregnancy.

Cooking and eating during pregnancy should be *fun and easy*. So enjoy reading this book; once you're done, throw together the recipe ingredients and dig in!

Radha McLean

THE GREEN PREGNANCY DIET:
WHAT IT MEANS AND HOW TO DO IT

You have probably never heard of a green pregnancy diet and may be suspicious of any phrase that places the word *diet* next to the word *pregnancy*. So what is a green pregnancy diet? First of all, eating green is far removed from the common perception of a diet; it has nothing to do with weight loss or restricting you from eating healthy amounts of nutritious food. What it does mean is that you can optimize your diet—eat the best that you possibly can—in the interest of having a healthy pregnancy, giving birth to a healthy baby and protecting the planet to boot.

HOW CAN I EAT GREEN DURING MY PREGNANCY?

Eating green focuses on consuming nutritious food without added chemicals and hormones, and avoiding those that cause the most harm to the planet. By creating a green diet for yourself in the crucial, precious months before your baby arrives, you'll not only provide the best possible nutrition for you and your baby, but you'll make a positive impact on the world for future generations.

EATING ORGANIC—BETTER FOR YOU, YOUR BABY, AND THE PLANET

The first and arguably biggest step you can take toward having a green diet is to eat organic food. Organic food, most commonly in the form of dairy products, fruits and vegetables, is becoming increasingly popular, especially during pregnancy. Take a look at the reasons why.

DEFINING ORGANIC FOOD

The U.S. Department of Agriculture (USDA) defines organic food as that which is "produced by farmers who emphasize the use of renewable resources and the conservation of soil and water to enhance environmental quality for future generations. Organic meat, poultry, eggs, and dairy products come from animals that are given no antibiotics or growth hormones. Organic food is produced without using most conventional pesticides."[1]

NONORGANIC FOOD AND HEALTH

As described above, since the mid-twentieth century, conventionally grown (nonorganic) fruits, vegetables, grains, and beans have been grown using pesticides and herbicides. Pesticides and herbicides are toxic chemicals used to control insects, rodents, weeds, mold, fungus, and bacteria. Exposure to these chemicals has been shown to increase the risk of a host of health conditions and diseases, including breast cancer and non-Hodgkin's lymphoma, among other cancers.[2] By eating conventionally grown foods during your pregnancy, you expose both yourself and your baby to these harmful toxins.

NONORGANIC FOOD AND THE PLANET

Global warming is hitting us hard in more ways than we can wrap our heads around, from poor air and water quality to massive droughts and natural disasters across the globe. What does food have to do with the global warming? Conventionally grown foods are grown using toxic chemicals that pollute the air, water, and ground, and use more energy—mainly gas and fossil fuels—to produce than organic food.

So it benefits you, your baby and the planet to go organic as much as possible.

ORGANIC FOOD IS HARD TO FIND AND EXPENSIVE. WHAT CAN I DO?

It may be hard to go completely organic. Organic food can be more expensive and is not always available at a nearby store. The organic versions of some common foods, however, are similar in price to nonorganic counterparts and commonly sold in stores. These foods include dairy (milk and cheese) and everyday fruits (apples and bananas).

Also, the availability of organic foods is increasing in general, so it's easier to find organic options today than it was in the past. For a start, farmers markets and major supermarket chains have started carrying organic foods. What's more, in major cities such as New York, online supermarkets with organic items will deliver to your door. There are even organic farms, community-supported agriculture programs and online stores dedicated exclusively to organic food, which provide online ordering and home delivery in some areas. For a list of some farmers' markets and online stores with organic products, check out the Resources chapter at the end of this book.

The organic dairy, fruit, and vegetables used in the recipes in this book are now sold in many grocery stores and supermarkets. Consider buying organic soy, beans, rice, pasta, bread and more if you can find them.

EATING VEGETARIAN FOOD
—THE REASONS WHY PEOPLE DO IT

Many women choose not to eat meat, fish or dairy for periods of time or in general for many reasons. Some opt for a full-time vegetarian or vegan diet for health, environmental or ethical reasons, or personal preference. Others may be part-time vegetarians: flexitarians (who eat vegetarian foods at home but don't resist the occasional burger), pescetarians (who hate red meat but *love* fish) or equal opportunity eaters (who love veggies and steak alike!).

On the other hand, some women may avoid meat or fish—or both—only after becoming pregnant. Some mothers simply can't stomach the thought of swallowing that chicken sandwich between bouts of morning sickness. Others skip animal sources of food during pregnancy to avoid potentially harmful additives in fish and meat, or to refrain from contributing to planet warming caused by large-scale fish and meat production.

FISH AND HEALTH

Many common types of fish, which are otherwise great sources of certain nutrients like protein and omega-3 fats, contain mercury. Mercury has been shown to be associated with premature birth,autism,and lower cognition in the children of mothers who had high levels of it in their bodies during pregnancy. [3,4,5]

For this reason, a Food and Drug Administration (FDA) advisory on mercury states that pregnant women and women who could become pregnant should eat no more than 12 ounces of fish a week.[6] If you choose to eat fish before or while you're pregnant, or you have a child and are giving that child fish to eat, experts recommend eating fish low in mercury, which include anchovies, Atlantic herring, wild and farmed salmon, sardines and trout. You can also get a list of the types of fish with low mercury and those that are not in risk of extinction online from Natural Resources Defense Council (www.nrdc.org/health/ effects/mercury/guide.asp).[7] If you eat local fish, check the U.S. Environmental Protection Agency's Web site for local advisories in your state that tell you which types of local fish are safe to eat (www.epa.gov/waterscience/fish/ states.htm).[8]

Another health concern from eating fish is the potential chemicals found in fish grown at fish farms. These fish may be exposed to medications, pesticides, herbicides and/or genetic engineering.[9]

FISH AND THE PLANET

From an environmental point of view, eating certain types of fish also contributes in a notable way to global warming. The majority of fish sold in the United States are imported, which means that large amounts of gas and oil are used for their transportation. Of the fish that are not imported, those that come from fish farming use massive amounts of water (four hundred gallons of water for one pound of fish), food, and electricity to produce.[9]

MEAT AND HEALTH

The cattle used for nonorganic dairy and meat poses a threat to a pregnant woman's health as well. Nonorganic cattle may be fed antibiotics and/or a steroid called recombinant bovine growth hormone. Bovine growth hormone is given to increase milk production and muscle mass. Giving cattle this hormone may cause them to produce extra amounts of another hormone, called insulin-like growth factor-1. Studies have shown that insulin-like growth factor-1 found in meat contributes to the development of breast cancer.[10] For this reason, hormonal additives in meat are banned in Europe and Canada, even though they are still allowed in the United States.

The Environmental Working Group (www.ewg.org), a not-for-profit environmental research organization dedicated to improving public health and protecting the environment, recommends that you limit your exposure to hormones and pesticides, especially during pregnancy.

MEAT AND THE PLANET

Large-scale production of meat is a major cause of global warming. A recent report from United Nations Food and Agriculture Organization found that meat production accounts for 18 percent of global warming emissions worldwide, which is more than the amount of global warming caused by transportation.[11] Why? Millions of acres of forests are cleared to make space for large-scale cattle farming, which kills wildlife and damages the soil. Also, it takes massive amounts of food, water, and gas to feed, raise and transport animals bred for meat. Plus, animal manure, produced in large quantities as a byproduct of large-scale factory farming, emits the greenhouse gases methane and nitrous oxide into the air.

MAKING CHANGES TO YOUR DIET

All of the recipes in this book contain organic foods, and no meat or fish for these reasons—they're good for you, your baby and the planet!

Cutting out meat or fish, or both, may not be for you. If that's the case, do what you can when you're pregnant for the health benefits—stick with organic and/or locally produced meat when it's an option and limit your fish intake to 12 ounces a week. If you want to eat less meat for environmental reasons, literally every meal makes a difference. For example, if every American skipped one meal with chicken a week and substituted it with vegetables and grains, the carbon monoxide savings would equal taking more than half a million cars off of U.S. roads. Eating one meal without red meat a week would be the same as taking more than five million cars off our roads, and eating one meat-free day a week would mean taking eight million cars off American roads.[12]

This concept is not far from the mainstream. An article in the *New York Times* acknowledges the multiple reasons for eating less meat without cutting it out altogether, and gives some tips for how to go about doing it—one of which is to dismiss the idea that you cannot get enough protein without eating meat, since plenty of plant foods are high in protein.[13]

HEAVY METAL DETOXIFICATION

If you're not pregnant *and* not trying yet, consider undergoing a heavy metal detoxification program.

Detoxification, or detox, will help rid your body of any heavy metals such as lead and mercury that may have built up over the years from eating foods with toxins like fish and nonorganic produce, and being exposed to environmental toxins in water, paint, air pollution and other sources. The first step in the detoxification process is to find a reputable naturopathic or medical doctor who specializes in heavy metal detox. This healthcare provider will first test you for high heavy metal levels using a urine test. Next, he or she will create a heavy metal detox program for you that may include one or more of the following components: supplements, herbal teas, juices, exercise program, dietary plan, spa treatments and hot baths. A good resource for finding a trusted naturopathic doctor is the American Association of Naturopathic Physicians (http://www.naturopathic.org).

Do not, however, consider detoxifying if you're already pregnant. This process could remove important minerals from your body and expose your growing baby to released toxins that have been stored in your body. Once you're pregnant, focus on getting the right amounts of the nutrients you need.

DIETARY ADVICE

If you want dietary advice in preparation for or during your pregnancy, ask your primary care provider for help and consider seeing a dietician. You can find a certified dietitian in your area from the American Dietetic Association (www.eatright.org).

2

NUTRITION DURING YOUR PREGNANCY: CHOOSING HEALTHY FOODS

Choosing a healthy diet is simple: eat grains, vegetables, fruits, protein and healthy fats, in that order, from largest to smallest servings. The same concept applies to your diet during pregnancy. The only difference is that it's perfectly okay—in fact, it's essential—that you eat more of certain nutrients once you're pregnant. Why? Because your body needs more energy and nutrients to support the growth of your baby.

> **WHAT NUTRIENTS ARE IMPORTANT TO GET DURING MY PREGNANCY, AND HOW MUCH OF EACH NUTRIENT SHOULD I GET EVERY DAY?**

While you know it's important to eat well, getting a grasp on the different nutrients a pregnant woman needs and making sure you get the right amounts each day may seem daunting. The information and tables to follow explain all the nutrients you need, how much of each one you should get daily, and how to get the right amounts from food and supplements.

Pregnant women need to get more of certain nutrients than they did before pregnancy because the amounts of these nutrients in the body changes during pregnancy. These items include folic acid, protein, vitamin B_{12} and others. On the other hand, the amount of calcium and eight lesser known nutrients you need doesn't change during pregnancy (see Table 1 for a complete list of the nutrients).[14]

CAN I GET ALL THE NUTRIENTS I NEED IF I CUT BACK OR ELIMINATE FISH OR MEAT FROM MY DIET?

If you want to avoid fish and/or meat or just cut back on these foods during your pregnancy, it is safe to do so. If your loved ones want proof, you can tell them that, when providing dietary recommendations during pregnancy, the American Dietetic Association and USDA both place beans, legumes and nuts in the same food group as meat and allow meat to be replaced by these plant sources.[15,16] The information and recipes in this book can be enjoyed by every type of vegetarian-friendly woman—from vegans to the equal opportunity eaters.

The key to eating a healthy diet during this precious and crucial time is to be informed about the nutrients you need and *get them from food sources and supplements*. The major nutrients most commonly found in meat, fish and dairy include iron, B_{12}, zinc, protein, and omega-3 fats. There are plenty of vegetarian sources of protein, zinc and iron, while omega-3 fats are harder to get (one type is only found in fish and algae), and B_{12} is found in dairy but not in plant sources.

Table 1. Recommended daily amounts of nutrients before and during pregnancy[14]

Nutrient	Before Pregnancy	During Pregnancy
nutrients that change		
Vitamin A	700 mcg	770 mcg
Vitamin C	75 mg	85 mg
Thiamin	1.1 mg	1.4 mg
Riboflavin	1.1 mg	1.4 mg
Niacin	14 mg	18 mg
Vitamin B$_6$	1.3 mg	1.9 mg
Folic Acid	400 mcg	600 mcg
Vitamin B$_{12}$	2.4 mcg	2.6 mcg
Pantothenic acid	2.4 mcg	2.6 mcg
Choline	425 mg	450 mg
Chromium	25 mcg	30 mcg
Copper	900 mcg	1000 mcg
Iodine	150 mcg	220 mcg
Iron	18 mg	27 mg
Magnesium	310 mg (19–30 years old); 320 (31–50 years old)	350 mg (19–30 years old); 360 (31–50 years old)
Manganese	1.8 mg	2.0 mg
Molybdenum	45 mcg	50 mcg
DHA	220 mg	300 mg
Selenium	55 mcg	60 mcg
Zinc	8 mg	11 mg
Water	2.7 liters	3 liters
Carbohydrates (minimum)	130 mg	175 mg
Fiber	25 g	28 g
Linoleic acid	12 g	18 g
ALA	1.1 g	1.4 g
Protein	46 g	71 g
nutrients that do not change		
EPA	220 mg	220 mg
Vitamin D	5 mcg (200 IU)	5 mcg (200 IU)
Vitamin E	15 mg	15 mg
Vitamin K	90 mcg	90 mcg
Biotin	30 mcg	30 mcg
Calcium	1000 mg	1000 mg
Phosphorus	700 mg	700 mg
Potassium	4.7 g	4.7 g
Chloride	2.3 g	2.3 g

A WORD ABOUT SERVING SIZES

The USDA uses the term *serving* to define the amount of each food group you should eat daily. But one serving can be confusing, especially when you are told by the USDA to eat six to eight servings a day.[16] Most of you don't eat six to eight times per day, nor do you limit yourself to eating one serving in each meal.

A real-life translation of servings is to measure meals in cups. For example, an average-sized dinner usually has one cup of grain such as bread, pasta or rice (two servings), and one half cup of legumes or beans (two servings).

Table 2 lists the daily serving sizes in cups for each food group, the number of servings you should get a day, and examples of food amounts that equal one serving. The right number of servings for you varies based on your due date, height, weight, age and amount of exercise. Check out the USDA's personalized food guidelines for pregnancy, which is called My Pyramid, on the Web (www.mypyramid.gov/mypyramidmoms/index.html).[16] You can easily calculate a personalized diet plan based on your demographics.

Table 2: Daily recommended amount of each food group during pregnancy[16]*

Group	Servings a day	Portion equal to number of servings
Grains, bread, rice and pasta (measured in ounces or ounce equivalents) Recommended that half of total comes from whole grains	6–10 servings (ounces)	One serving: 1 slice of bread; 1/2 cup of cooked grains (oatmeal, rice, pasta, etc.); 1 cup of ready-to-eat cereal; 5 whole wheat crackers; 1 small pancake Three servings: 1 muffin Four servings: 1 microwave bag popcorn, 1 large tortilla, 1 large bagel
Vegetables	2.5–4 servings (cups)	One serving: 2 cups raw leafy vegetables; 1 cup of cooked vegetables; 1 medium potato; 1 cup of vegetable juice
Fruits	1.5 –2.5 servings (cups)	1 piece of fruit; 1 cup chopped fruit; 1/2 cup dried fruit; 1 cup of fruit juice

Group	Servings a day	Portion equal to number of servings
Milk, yogurt and cheese (measured in cups)	3 cups	One serving: 1 cup of milk or yogurt; 1/3 cup (1 1/2 ounces) natural (unprocessed) cheese; 1/2 cup (2 ounces) processed American cheese; 2 cups cottage cheese; 1 cup calcium fortified soy milk
Legumes, beans, eggs, and nuts*	5–7 servings (ounces)	One serving: 1/4 cup of cooked beans (black, kidney, pinto, garbanzo, lentils, etc.); 1 egg; 1/4 cup of tofu; 2 Tbsp hummus; 1/3 cup (1/2 oz) nuts (12 almonds, 24 pistachios or 7 walnut halves); 1 Tbsp peanut butter Two servings: 1/4 cup (2 oz) cooked tempeh

*Meat, poultry and fish have been excluded in this table from the USDA's protein food group.

WHAT FOODS HAVE THE MAJOR NUTRIENTS I NEED, AND WHERE CAN I FIND THEM?

The food sources for each major nutrient and how much nutrient is found in one portion are shown in Table 3. A lot of these foods are included in the recipes in this book, and you are reminded in the recipes of the foods' nutritional values (so don't worry, you won't be tested!).

VITAMINS AND MINERALS

CALCIUM

Calcium is important for both mommy and baby because it is the building block for bones and teeth and helps keep bones strong. Although it's important to get calcium, you don't require more calcium during pregnancy. Women aged 19–50—pregnant or not—need 1,000 mg of calcium per day.[17] (Teenaged girls aged 9–13 need more—1,300 mg daily.[17]) Calcium can be found in abundance in beans, legumes, nuts, fruit and, dairy.[18] See Table 3 for types of foods and amounts of calcium in each food.[19]

FOLIC ACID

Folic acid, or folate, is fundamental to the function and repair of cells in your body. Low amounts of folic acid in the diet have been linked to birth defects, making it a critical nutrient in your diet even before you become pregnant. The Recommended Dietary Allowance of folic acid while pregnant is 600 micrograms (mcg) a day.[16] While you can get folic acid from greens, beans, citrus fruit, and whole fortified wheat bread, your healthcare provider will recommend taking a prenatal vitamin daily during your pregnancy to get your daily amount. In fact, it's important to start getting the daily recommended amount before pregnancy since folic acid helps form the baby's spinal cord, which develops early in pregnancy.

If you're pregnant and haven't started taking a folic acid supplement, don't fret, but do buy a daily prenatal supplement right away! A prenatal vitamin will give you a lot of your daily intake of folic acid. But that shouldn't stop you from getting as much as you can in your diet from foods. Folic acid is found in grains, beans, vegetables and fruits (see Table 3 for details).

IRON

Iron carries oxygen in the blood, so it is essential for your body's function and development. Pregnant women should get at least 27 mg of iron a day. While the Centers for Disease Control and Prevention recommend taking an iron supplement, you'll get all the iron you need from your prenatal vitamin and by eating foods with iron in them.[20] Since an iron supplement often causes constipation, many women prefer not to take one.

There are two types of iron: heme iron, found in meat and absorbed better by the body, and nonheme iron, found in plant foods and not absorbed as well. Although meat is high in the kind of iron that is better absorbed, you can easily get all the iron you need during pregnancy without the meat—by eating plant foods high in iron (see Table 3 for food ideas) and taking a prenatal vitamin that contains iron.

Your body absorbs iron better if it is eaten with foods that have vitamin C; so try to combine your high iron foods with those that have vitamin C. Some good sources of vitamin C are potatoes, broccoli, tomatoes, peppers (red, yellow, and orange), oranges, papaya, mangos, and kiwi fruit.

It's also helpful to know that certain compounds do the opposite of vitamin C—they stop the absorption of iron. These compounds include the oxalic acid found in spinach and chocolate, tannins in tea and coffee, phytates in beans, and polyphenols in coffee. It's not a big deal—just avoid eating these items when you eat iron-rich foods. Or, eat your iron-rich food (beans) and absorption-preventing food (beans) with a vitamin C-containing food (potatoes, broccoli or peppers).

VITAMIN B₁₂

Vitamin B_{12} is also essential for the growth of your baby; it supports healthy nerve and red blood cells and helps create DNA, one of the building blocks of all cells. The daily recommended amount during pregnancy is 2.6 mcg.[14] B_{12}, included in prenatal vitamins, is also found in abundance in meat and dairy. If you are following a vegetarian diet, make sure you eat some dairy and that your prenatal vitamin contains vitamin B_{12}. Those of you who don't eat dairy, however, must track your B_{12} intake every day. Non-animal sources of the vitamin are found in fortified cereals, soymilk and, soy products, nutritional yeast and prenatal vitamins (see Table 3).

ZINC

Zinc, an important mineral that supports biochemical reactions and a healthy immune system, is used for tissue growth and repair and is one of more than two hundred enzymes. Deficiency of zinc can cause birth defects, so it's important that you get enough zinc during your pregnancy. The daily recommended amount of zinc goes up from 8 to 11 mg in pregnancy.[16] While animal protein offers the highest source of zinc, a prenatal vitamin will have the right amount. You can also get high amounts of zinc from wheat germ and smaller amounts from other plant foods and dairy (see Table 3).

WHAT ABOUT CALORIES, FAT AND PROTEIN— ISN'T IT IMPORTANT TO PAY ATTENTION TO HOW MUCH I EAT DAILY?

A host of elements other than vitamins and minerals compose the food we eat. While these elements are important sources of nutrients and energy for your body, some of these nutrients include foods with poor nutrition and added toxins.

OTHER ELEMENTS IN FOOD

CALORIES

Calories represent the energy in the food you eat—the sum total of the nutrients and other elements discussed in this chapter. You need a certain amount of energy to function on a healthy level. It's a given, however, that if you eat too much, you'll consume too many calories (that is, too much energy), which can lead to unnecessary weight gain and other health problems during pregnancy.

Some diets and eating plans base their recommendations on calorie intake, otherwise known as "counting calories." The information and recipes in this book focus on meeting the specific nutritional needs during your pregnancy, so counting calories will not be discussed. The Institute of Medicine (IOM), which provides dietary guidelines for all Americans, does not count calories either; rather, they establish a healthy range for how much fat, carbohydrates and protein you should be eating daily.[21]

Table 3. Major nutrients and food sources (ranked by most to least grams)[19]

Nutrient	Food Group	Food	Portion	Amount/nutrient
Calcium	Dairy	Milk or yogurt	1 cup	300 mg
		Cheese	1 cup	300 mg
	Beans	Soy (soy yogurt, cooked or dry roasted soybeans, tofu, tempeh and fortified soymilk)	1/2 cup	100–400 mg
		Cooked black, kidney and garbanzo beans	1/2 cup	40–60 mg
	Nuts and seeds	Sesame seeds	2 Tbsp tahini	130 mg

Nutrient	Food Group	Food	Portion	Amount/nutrient
Calcium		Almonds	1/4 cup almonds or 2 Tbsp almond butter	90 mg
	Fruit	Figs	5 dried	approx. 140 mg
		Orange	1 large orange or 1/2 cup juice	75 mg–150 mg
	Vegetables	Bok choy, collard greens and turnips	1 cup cooked	100–200 mg
Folic Acid	Grains	Enriched and fortified bread, rice, flour and breakfast cereals	1 cup	Up to 400 mcg

Nutrient	Category	Food	Amount	Content
Folic Acid	Beans	Most types of beans, including soy	1 cup	150–300 mcg
	Vegetables	Spinach and asparagus	1 cup	250 mcg
		Wheat germ	1/4 cup	100 mcg
		Broccoli	1 cup	50 mcg
		Avocado	1/2 avocado	80 mcg
	Fruit	Orange juice	1 cup	75–110 mcg
	Grains	Fortified whole grain cold breakfast cereal	1 cup	Up to 18 mg
Iron		Cream of Wheat	1 cup	8 mg

Nutrient	Food Group	Food	Portion	Amount/nutrient
Iron		Fortified instant oatmeal	1 cup	4 mg
		Whole grain cold breakfast cereal	1 cup	At least 2 mg
		Wheat germ	2 Tbsp	1 mg
		Bread	1 slice	.5–1 mg
		Enriched rice	1/2 cup	1.4 mg
		Pumpkin and squash seeds	1/4 cup	8 mg
	Nuts and seeds	Cashews, sunflower seeds	1/4 cup	2–2.3 mg

Iron				
		Tahini (sesame seeds)	2 Tbsp	2.7
	Beans	Cooked soy beans	1/2 cup	4.4 mg
		Tofu	1/2 cup	3.4 mg
		Most types of beans other than soy	1/2 cup	2–3 mg
		Dry roasted soybeans, soymilk, tempeh	1/2 cup	.4 to 2 mg
	Fruit	Prune juice	3/4 cup	2.3 mg

Nutrient	Food Group	Food	Portion	Amount/nutrient
	Vegetables	Apricots (dried), currants, figs, prunes, raisins	1/4–1/2 cup	.5–1 mg
		Baked potato with skin	1	more than 2 mg
		Most vegetables	1/2 cup	almost 1 mg
	Dairy	Egg yolk	1	.9 mg
Zinc	Grains	Wheat germ	1/4 cup	4.7 mg
		Bread	1 slice	.5 mg
	Nuts and Seeds	Sunflower seeds	1/4 cup	2 mg

	Category	Food	Serving	Amount
	Beans	Most types of beans, including soy	1/2 cup	1–2 mg
	Dairy	Milk	1 cup	1 mg
		Eggs	1	.6 mg
ALA	Nuts and seeds	Flaxseed oil, whole or ground flaxseeds	1 Tbsp	Up to 7 g
		Walnuts, walnut oil	1/4 cup	1.5–2.9 g
		Hemp seed, hemp seed nut butter	1 Tbsp	2 g
	Grains	Uncle Sam cereal	1 cup	3.3 g

Nutrient	Food Group	Food	Portion	Amount/nutrient
ALA	Oil	Perilla	1 tsp	3 g
		Canola	1 Tbsp	1.5 g
	Beans	Soy beans, tofu	1/2 cup	500–700 mg
		Pinto	1 cup	400 mg
		ALA-enriched soy milk	1 cup	400 mg
	Vegetables	Canned grape leaves	1/3 cup (2 oz)	480 mg
Protein	Dairy	Cheese	1/4 cup (2 oz)	12–14 g
		Yogurt	1 small container (8 oz)	10 g

Protein			
	Milk	1 cup	8 g
Beans	Soymilk	1 cup	8 g
	Tofu, firm	1/4 cup (81 grams or 1/4 block)	6 g
	Soy-based fake meat	Varies; see package label for serving size	Varies; see package label for amount
	Most other beans	1/2 cup	6–9 g
	Most nuts	1/4 cup (1 oz)	6 g
Nuts	Peanut butter	1 Tbsp	4 g
Grains	Cooked quinoa	1 cup	8 g

Nutrient	Food Group	Food	Portion	Amount/nutrient
Protein		Cooked buckwheat groats	1 cup	6 g
		Bread	1 slice	4 g
		Cold breakfast cereal	1 cup	2–5 g
	Vegetables	Sweet potato	1 cup	3 g
		Green veggies	½ cup	2-3 g
	Fruit	Most types of fruit	1 cup whole or juice	2 g or less

If you want to know your calorie intake, you will find the number of calories per serving in the recipes provided in this book.

CARBOHYDRATES

Carbohydrates, or carbs, are essential for giving your body energy. How many carbs should you be eating a day? Rather than "counting carbs," pregnant women should focus on eating the recommended number of servings in each of the five food groups—all of which contain carbs. The recommended amount of carbs to eat daily during your pregnancy is 175 mg, as mentioned in Table 1.[16]

A low-carb diet is not an option during pregnancy; it poses a risk to your baby's brain and body development. Yet, eating too many carbs can be a problem as well—one far too common in diets today. The servings of breads, cereals, grains, legumes, fruits, and vegetables that we eat with every meal provide all the carbs we need, but we often eat more carbs a day than we should. (Let's admit it—they taste good!). Yet, some of this excess carb intake is unintentional, as described below.

Carbs are made up of simple carbs (fruit, dairy, and sugars) and complex carbs (beans, grains, legumes, nuts, and vegetables).

SIMPLE CARBS

Sugar is the main component of simple carbs, and can be defined by sugars found naturally in food and those that are added to food.

Sugar found naturally in food: You may have heard of the Glycemic Index (GI). The concept is simple. Most foods contain sugar, and the GI measures how much of that food converts into glucose (or body sugar) when you eat it. Whole fruit and milk are the simple carbs that contain some natural sugars but do not have high GIs. On the opposite end, processed sugars like fruit juice and refined sugars like "white" (cane) sugar have sky high GIs. So they convert to high levels of glucose after we eat them because a lot of the fiber, minerals, and vitamins have been removed. It goes without saying that simple carbs with a lower GI are less "sugary" and therefore generally better for you.

Sugars added to food: Because most of the food we eat already contains natural forms of sugar, there is no health benefit to adding sugars or sweeteners to food. Added sugars have high GIs and contain a lot of calories. The problem, however, is that it's easy to overlook the added sugar in foods and to end up eating too much. For example, if you've eaten sugar-sweetened cereal for breakfast and a cookie as a snack, you've likely packed in more sugar than your body needs for the day without realizing it—and all before eating your lunch, dinner and bedtime snack.

One of the reasons it's so hard to avoid sugar is because it's added to so many of the foods that we eat regularly—not just dessert. You'll be amazed, once you take close look at food labels, how much sugar is added to otherwise healthy prepared foods like yogurt and cold breakfast cereal. Sugar is also added to bread, snack bars, jelly, peanut butter, canned fruits, and vegetables, ketchup, salad dressings, and tomato sauce—the list goes on and on.

There is good news. You can find some of these foods *without* added sugar. Buy unsweetened yogurt, jelly, peanut butter, and canned fruits and vegetables whenever possible. This means you'll have to read the list of ingredients and sugar contents on labels the next time you go grocery shopping. Once you've pinned down the brands without sugar, you can head straight for them next time, and buying sugar-free foods will no longer seem like a chore.

Certain foods, however, are almost impossible to find unsweetened, such as breakfast cereal, ketchup and desserts. If an unsweetened option is not available, avoid buying foods with the following, less healthy, refined forms of sugar:

- white (refined cane) sugar
- corn syrup or high fructose corn syrup

Look for brands of foods sweetened with these healthier, unrefined forms of sugar:

- barley malt syrup
- brown rice syrup
- date sugar
- fruit juice
- honey
- maple syrup
- molasses
- whole fruit

These sweeteners are healthier for you than white sugar and corn syrup because they contain more nutrients and are processed without using toxic chemicals. Also, most natural sweeteners have lower GIs than refined sugars, so they're less fattening and challenging for your kidneys to process. *Please note that agave, a natural sweetener taken from the agave plant that has recently been appearing on store shelves, should not be eaten during pregnancy since it may be associated with birth defects.*

Even if a healthier sweetener such as honey is the first ingredient listed on a label, it means that it is the most prevalent ingredient. This is a bad sign. Try to find another food item in which the sweetener is listed farther down in the list of ingredients. Also, look at the total grams of sugar in a serving to find out how much sugar has been added. Go for the brand with the lowest number of grams of sugar whenever possible.

Additive sweeteners: Additive sweeteners—commonly in the form of artificial sweeteners and colors and sugar replacements—are other extras added to some foods to enhance or preserve the appearance, sweetness and/or flavor. Some common additive sweeteners you may have seen on food labels include these:

- Aspartame
- Equal
- NutraSweet
- Organic Zero
- Saccharin
- Splenda
- Stevia

Many of these products are processed with chemicals, which place toxins in your bloodstream that could then be transferred to your baby. *Further, it is not known whether or not these sweeteners are safe to eat during pregnancy, so try to avoid this list of additives completely.*

Yes, that means avoiding artificially-flavored diet soda! If you normally drink carbonated sodas or crave them during your pregnancy, try a natural brand. While some natural sodas contain unrefined cane sugar, they're a lesser evil than those made with artificial additives. Look for fruit-juice-sweetened soda or carbonated sparkling juice. Some all-natural brands of carbonated drinks can be found in the Resources chapter.

COMPLEX CARBS

Complex carbs include beans, grains, legumes, and vegetables. Grains are the most common source of complex carbs and can be found in two forms—whole grains and refined grains.

Whole grains are grains that have not been refined, leaving all three parts of the grain (bran, endosperm, and germ) intact.

The more common types of grains are refined grains. These grains have had most of their valuable nutrients removed during the refining process. *They are left with less fiber, few vitamins and minerals not to mention much higher GIs.* What about that is good for you? (Certain enriched refined grains have some nutrients, like folic acid, added back in.).

The most common refined grains are "white" (refined wheat) flour used to make bread and pasta and "white" (refined) rice. In fact, they're so common that you have to seek out the whole grain versions. Other grains, like corn, buckwheat, and oatmeal, are not generally refined. So if you see corn chips, soba noodles (made from buckwheat and whole wheat) or oatmeal bars at the supermarket, most likely the grain is in its nutritious form.

If you are ever unsure if a grain is a whole grain, it probably is not. For example, European breads like baguette and focaccia, and comfort foods such as white bread and the macaroni in "mac and cheese" are usually made with white flour. Bummer! Check prepared food labels for the phrases *multigrain, whole grain* or *whole wheat* to ensure that you are eating the healthier form of grain. To add variety to your diet, additional types of whole grains include amaranth, quinoa, millet, spelt, teff, and barley.

Beans, legumes, nuts, and vegetables contain some of the lowest levels of sugar of the complex carbs. As a general rule, eat healthier complex carbs—whole (unrefined) grains, vegetables, beans and legumes—as much as possible. Whole grains and other complex carbs are used in all of the recipes in this book.

PROTEIN

Protein provides you and your baby with the essential amino acids that make cells function. The amount of protein you should eat daily increases significantly when you're pregnant; from 46 grams a day to 71 grams a day.[14] It is vital that you track your protein intake to make sure you're getting enough protein during your pregnancy. (Hint: You should include some protein in every meal.) Protein can be found in abundance in meat and fish, but is also found in plenty of plant foods, including beans, grains, nuts, some fruits and vegetables, and in dairy. (See Table 3 for ideas.)

FIBER

Fiber is the part of a plant food that is used by your body for cell growth, energy, and much more. Fiber is not digested, and therefore it comes out in bodily waste. The benefits of a high-fiber diet are many, including the prevention of heart disease, cancer, diabetes, and obesity.

The daily recommended amount of fiber for women is 25 grams. This amount increases to 28 grams a day during pregnancy.[14] Fiber is most commonly found in whole grains, legumes, fruit, and vegetables. You may also want to know that the iron in your prenatal vitamin can cause constipation during pregnancy. Lots of fiber helps prevent this problem—all the more reason to eat lots of it!

FATS

IOM guidelines state that you should be getting 20 percent to 35 percent of your calories, or energy, from fat.[21] However, no one wants to get bogged down by calculating percentages to figure out how much fat you ate today, especially not while you're pregnant with a hungry, growing baby. The less formal approach to eating fat is simple: Eat the good fat, not the bad, following the daily recommended amounts found in Table 1.

FAT AND YOUR DIET—THE GOOD AND THE BAD

How do you know which fats are good for you and which are not? The four main types of fats are broken down into the following categories:

Saturated fats are found in red meat, dairy, chocolate (all chocolate, not just dark chocolate), salmon, eggs, coconut oil, and palm kernel oil. Diets high in this type of fat have been associated with heart disease. Generally, this category is considered "bad" fat.

Trans fats are fats taken from plant oils that have been altered to make them last longer and help keep food from spoiling. Trans fats are most commonly found in packaged baked goods, margarine, and fried foods. This type of fat has been shown to increase cholesterol and the risk of heart disease. This category is definitely considered "bad" fat!

Monounsaturated fats are found in nuts, avocados, whole wheat products, breakfast cereals, oatmeal, and most types of oil. These fats have been shown to protect against heart disease. But they may be associated with insulin resistance, which can lead to diabetes, so should be eaten in according to daily recommended amounts. This category is considered "good" fat.

Polyunsaturated fats are found in algae, fish, whole wheat products, breakfast cereal, peanut butter, most types of margarine, and sunflower and hemp seeds. Polyunsaturated fats are fundamental to brain and nerve development and function, in addition to lowering cholesterol. However, too much of them could be harmful. This category is certainly a "good" fat when consumed in the daily recommended amounts.

As you can see, good (monounsaturated and polyunsaturated) fats found in algae and fish are also found in plant sources, such as certain nuts, grains, seeds and fruit. While whole milk dairy products are rich in protein, calcium, and B vitamins, they are also high in bad (saturated) fat. For this reason, try to choose low-fat (1% or skim is best) milk, cheese, and yogurt during your pregnancy. It goes without saying that red meat is not "green" for previously mentioned health and environmental reasons in chapter 1; add to that the fact that it's a source of bad (saturated) fat. Trans fat, the indisputably bad type of fat, is most commonly found in store- and restaurant-bought fried foods. Stay away from these items, which include potato chips and french fries, as much as possible.

One more thing worth knowing about fats, which applies to the "good" and "bad" fats in the form of oil, is that oil heated at high levels needed to fry foods releases cancer-causing toxins. So fried foods, even if they are prepared with a "good" fat like olive oil, should generally be avoided.

Omega-3 fats. Omega-3 fats are a group of three types of good (polyunsaturated) fat fundamental to your baby's brain development (translation: eating omega-3 fats during pregnancy will make your baby smart!). These fats include alpha-linolenic acid (ALA), eicosapentaenoic acid (EPA), and docosahexaenoic acid (DHA). ALA acts as the "parent" fat, which is converted by the body into EPA and DHA. EPA and DHA have a more direct effect on your baby's development: EPA promotes brain function, concentration and vision, while DHA is especially important because it is used to create your baby's brain structure.

The International Society for the Study of Fatty Acids and Lipids (SSFAL) recommends that you get 300 mg of DHA and 220 mg of EPA daily during pregnancy (pre-pregnancy levels are 220 mg for both), with a limit of no more than 10 percent of calories from DHA/EPA.[24] The daily recommended amount of ALA is 1,400 mg (1.4 grams).[14] *While ALA is easily found in certain seeds and oils (see Table 3), DHA can only be found in algae and fish.* As mentioned in chapter 1, healthcare experts recommend limiting your fish intake during pregnancy due to mercury and other contaminants found in fish.[23] If you eat some fish, fish sources of DHA with low mercury include anchovies, Atlantic herring, wild and farmed salmon, sardines, and trout.

How can you make sure that you're getting the daily recommended amount of DHA (300 mg)? Taking a DHA supplement is your best bet. DHA comes from sea algae, which is eaten by fish. So a fish-oil or algae-based supplement is equally beneficial depending on your dietary preference. Fish-oil-based supplements can easily be found at your local drugstore. An algae-based supplement is less common. Deva is one brand that sells an algae-based supplement, which you can order online. Contact information for Deva can be found in the Resources chapter.

Be sure to ask your doctor when to start taking the supplement. If you have a disorder involving bleeding, bruise easily, or are taking blood thinners, consult with your doctor before taking this supplement since DHA is a documented blood thinner. Most pregnant women should take a 200-mg supplement once daily. If you don't take a DHA supplement and don't eat fish during your pregnancy, experts recommend that you double the amount of ALA in your diet. One study showed that the babies of vegetarian moms who did not take a DHA supplement had less DHA in their blood than those of moms who ate some fish during pregnancy.[22]

A supplement should not stop you from building ALA into your diet. Just as with other nutrients, ALA is best absorbed when eaten in your diet. The richest plant form of ALA is flaxseeds, with 7 grams in a tablespoon. You can find and eat flaxseeds in many forms—the whole seeds, ground seeds or oil. Many of the recipes in this book use flaxseeds since they're an easy fix to get your daily amount of ALA (1.4 grams). To get the ALA, flaxseeds need to be split by either being ground or chewed. So buy ground flaxseeds or grind them in a hand-held grinder if you want to make sure you get the full benefit of ALA. *However, you should not eat more than 4 grams of flaxseeds a day when you're pregnant since the effects of large amounts of flaxseeds have not been studied in pregnant women.* Walnuts are another great food source of ALA; however, walnuts are high in an amino acid called arginine, which can cause a herpes simplex virus outbreak. So women with the condition should avoid walnuts if it triggers an outbreak. These and more good plant sources of ALA can be found in Table 3.

SALT

Sodium, commonly eaten in the form of salt, is needed for the balance of fluids and for nerve and muscle activity in our bodies. Getting enough salt, however, is rarely a concern today because salt is added to nearly all the packaged foods we eat, from canned soup to tomato sauce. Further, some salt is found naturally in some plant foods such as broccoli and celery.

In reality, most of us need not be concerned about getting enough salt; instead, we should avoid eating too much since a high-salt diet can cause hypertension, diabetes, and kidney disease. If you currently have at least one of these conditions, consult with your healthcare professional or a dietitian immediately to develop a diet plan with the right amount of salt for you.

Even if you don't have one of these conditions, you may not be in the clear; salt causes your body to retain more water. This can lead to high blood pressure during pregnancy, even for women who had no blood pressure problems before becoming pregnant. So keep your daily intake of salt under the U.S. daily recommended limit of 2,400 mg (2.4 grams).[25]

FOOD SAFETY

The issue of food safety—something you may not have thought of before—comes into play when you're pregnant. Bacteria grow in certain types of raw and cold food, which can cause an infection called *listeriosis* when eaten. Listeriosis is life threatening for your baby—it can lead to miscarriage, stillbirth, premature delivery or infection of your newborn.

The Centers for Disease Control and Prevention recommend following these precautions to avoid getting a bacterial infection from food during pregnancy:[26]

- Do not eat the following foods raw: dairy, include raw cheeses, milk and eggs, fish, poultry, and meat.
- Do not eat any prepared meats, including hot dogs and deli meat.
- Heat/cook all leftover food well.
- Wash all fruits and vegetables before eating them.
- Wash your hands and utensils after handling uncooked food.
- Eat perishable foods as soon as possible.

FOOD ALLERGIES

As a final note, avoid eating foods that you're allergic to —whether they be dairy, gluten, nuts, wheat or another food—as an important part of optimizing your health when you're pregnant. If you think you'll be missing out on important nutrients, think again. You can get the nutrients you need from other foods. For example, some nutrient-rich grains that you can eat instead of gluten and wheat include buckwheat, corn, quinoa, soy, and rice. Dairy alternatives include milk and cheese made from soy or rice, and soy nut and sunflower seed butter are good alternatives to peanut butter. The recipes in this book include many of these food alternatives.

If you have a food allergy, take the alternatives found in these recipes and incorporate them into your daily cooking and eating.

3

Your kitchen:
Making and keeping it green

Creating a kitchen space that is free of chemicals and toxins and cutting down on waste is fundamental to keeping you, your baby and the planet safe. Cooking and cleaning with nontoxic kitchen supplies, buying local, organic foods, managing your garbage and using clean water are just a few ways to make (and keep) your kitchen green.

Cooking and cleaning

Cooking and cleaning with nontoxic kitchen supplies is perhaps the most fundamental step in making your kitchen green. For example, did you know that aluminum and nonstick pans leach toxins into your food, and many kitchen cleaning supplies contain poison that you end up inhaling and eating? Here are a few basic changes you can make to create a nontoxic kitchen:

Replace:

- aluminum pots and cutlery and non-stick pots and pans with stainless steel and/or cast iron.
- conventional brands of dishwashing liquid, and floor, drain, oven, and window cleaners with chemical-free brands. Many of these brands are listed in the Resources chapter.

Avoid:

- cleaning products that contain phosphates, solvents, chlorine, genetically modified ingredients, animal-derived ingredients or petroleum.
- paper products with polyvinyl chloride (PVC) or chlorine.
- cleaning products that contain volatile organic compounds (VOCs). For more information on the VOCs that can be found in cleaning products, go to the Environmental Protection Agency's Web page on VOCs (www.epa.gov/iaq/voc.html).
- all cleaning supplies that state "caution," "danger," "poison" or "warning" on the labels.
- air fresheners and deodorizers.

Buy:

- cleaning products that are nontoxic, biodegradable, hypoallergenic, and plant-derived if possible.

The task of replacing all of these items in your kitchen may seem monumental—and expensive. Take it one step at a time by replacing one or two cooking and cleaning items every time you go shopping. Before you know it, your kitchen will be greener!

If you're feeling ambitious or just love the idea of purifying your kitchen, you can take this project to the next level and make your own cleaning supplies. It's easier than you think! Some everyday kitchen items such as dishwashing liquid, vinegar, baking soda, and lemon juice can be used to make all-purpose floor and window cleaner. Some Web sites with basic recipes for cleaning supplies can be found in the Resources chapter.

BUYING FOOD

In chapter 1, you read about the benefits of buying organic foods. Buying local produce—foods grown nearby that require no or less energy to transport—is another great way to keep a green kitchen. Many towns and cities have green markets or farmers' markets—small outdoor markets where nearby farmers, bakers, and food makers sell locally grown fruits, vegetables, baked goods, jams, juices, and more. Some farms sell their produce on site, while others even deliver.

Contact your local community centers and farms to get information about the locations of farms and local markets near you. The Organic Consumers Association (www.organicconsumers.org) and Local Harvest (www. localharvest.org) feature search engines that list farmers' markets, family farms, and other sources of sustainably grown food throughout the United States.

GARBAGE MANAGEMENT

Even if you have the best of intentions when it comes to going green, it's virtually impossible to avoid creating garbage in the kitchen. While ordering food from your favorite Chinese restaurant down the street means you're left with wasteful plastic containers, cooking food from scratch doesn't avoid the garbage dilemma either. Everything is sold in containers or wrapped/placed in plastic—from milk, pasta, and rice to fruits and vegetables. What you're left with after an inspired twenty minutes in the kitchen of chopping, measuring, and heating is a heap of containers, plastic bags, peels, and pits. What can you do to keep trash to a minimum?

COMPOSTING

The first thing you can do to recycle your food waste is composting. Composting involves storing certain plant materials, including some food scraps, in a dark, wet, and aerated place. Here, microbes and worms break down the waste into a nutrient-rich form of dirt that can then be added to houseplants and soil.

If you have a yard, you can set up a spot for composting outside. If not, there are methods for indoor composting. A number of composting Resources can be found on the Internet. One Web site, How to Compost (www.howtocompost.org) provides the basics for indoor and outdoor composting. If neither of these options works for you, you may be able to drop your compost material off at a local farmers' market or community garden. Some cities, such as San Francisco, have begun curbside compost collection services.

RECYCLING

Recycling is one of the most popular ways to keep your kitchen green. Some cities and towns pick up recycling outside your home, while others have recycling drop-off locations.

In most locations that recycle, all glass products and most metal and paper products can be recycled. Most types of plastics, on the other hand, cannot be recycled. Plastics are made in seven different ways. Most plastic products have diamond-shaped symbol made of arrows found on the bottom. Each symbol has a number, from 1 to 7, in the center. Plastic types 1 and 2 are most commonly recycled, while plastics 3–7 are harder to recycle.

Contact your local sanitation department to find out which ones they take and where your household products can be recycled in your area.

REUSING

Using ceramic dishes, metal cutlery, cloth napkins, and glass and safe plastic containers to store food, and reusing items you would otherwise throw away—such as plastic and paper shopping bags—are some additional ways that you can cut down on waste in the kitchen.

Not only do you add less garbage to landfills, but you save money, too—why buy disposable garbage bags when you can use bags you already have? Also, drugstores and supermarkets are starting to sell reusable canvas bags for shopping; these provide a fantastic way to cut down on waste. Reusing is a hard habit to start but an easy one to keep once you make it part of your routine.

When it comes to reusing plastic containers, it's important to check the numbers in the symbol on the bottom of the container since certain plastics have been shown to leach toxins. Plastics with the numbers 1, 2, 4, and 5 have not been shown to leach toxins. *Plastics with the numbers 3, 6, and 7, however, should be avoided for storing food since they could leach toxins into your food.* So no matter how committed you are to reusing, throw away all plastics in your kitchen with the numbers 3, 6, or 7 and avoid acquiring new ones when possible.

USING WATER IN THE KITCHEN

WATER FOR DRINKING

Remember when you used to drink water from the tap at your kitchen sink when you were growing up? In a single generation it seems as if we've gone from keeping it simple to making it complicated when it comes to the water we drink.

Sure, tap water is just as it was when you were a child. But concerns about increasing levels of minerals, pollution, toxins, and even trace amounts of prescription drugs in tap water, not to mention additives to drinking water like chlorine, leave us hesitant to drink that free cup at room temperature, especially during pregnancy. In response to these concerns, the sale bottled water that is marketed as cleaner than tap water has become a multi-million-dollar industry.

Some types of bottled water are, indeed, better than tap, while others are the same tap water disguised by packaging and a price tag, The FDA defines the different types of water:[27]

- Artesian well water comes from a well that taps an aquifer—layers of porous rock, sand and earth that contain water—which is under pressure from surrounding upper layers of rock or clay.
- Spring water is taken from an underground source where water flows naturally to the earth's surface.

- Mineral water comes from an underground source that contains at least 250 parts per million total dissolved solids. Minerals and trace elements must come from the source of the underground water. They cannot be added later.
- Well water comes from a hole bored or drilled into the ground, which taps into an aquifer.

Bottled water can come from "municipal sources"—in other words, before being bottled the tap water is usually treated in one of the following ways:

- Distillation. In this process, water is turned into a vapor. Since minerals are too heavy to vaporize, they are left behind, and the vapors are condensed into water again.
- Reverse osmosis. Water is forced through membranes to remove minerals in the water.
- Absolute 1 micron filtration. Water flows through filters that remove particles larger than 1 micron in size, such as *Cryptosporidium*, a parasite.
- Ozonation. Bottlers of all types of waters typically use ozone gas, an antimicrobial agent, instead of chlorine to disinfect the water.

Bottled water is water that has been treated by distillation, reverse osmosis or another suitable process and that meets the definition of "purified water" in the U.S. Pharmacopeia can be labeled as "purified water."

Some healthy skepticism is not a bad thing when it comes to paying a pretty penny to buy something that's available for free. So should you really be drinking water than is cleaner than tap water?

The short answer is: yes. The longer answer is: yes, but not necessarily by buying bottled water. Installing a high-end water filter system on your kitchen sink is possibly the most environmentally-friendly way to get chemical-free water. You're drinking the good stuff but without paying for each bottle and using disposable plastic containers. (Recycling plastic is less green than not using plastic at all—it takes a lot of energy and chemicals to recycle and frequently ends up in a landfill without being recycled).

A number of high-quality home filter systems are available, ranging in price. The Aquasana home water filter system, rated as number one by *Consumer Reports* five years in a row, is an affordable option. The down side of this system is that it uses plastic containers and tubes.

If you want to avoid using a plastic filter, Multipure has a system made of stainless steel that filters out the hard-to-remove toxins including mercury and asbestos. The higher end AKAI system uses ultraviolet rays to disinfect germs, bacteria, and viruses. Kangen, from Japan, is said to be perhaps the best water filter system on the market—it actually adds good minerals and antioxidants to the water, in addition to eliminating toxins and free radicals.

So do your research! You may decide that you want to invest in an expensive system, which will benefit you for decades to come. Keep in mind, however, that you should replace the filter regularly; otherwise, the benefits of the filter will diminish. Contact information for all of these water filters systems can be found in the Resources chapter.

WATER FOR COOKING

Heating water kills the unwanted bacteria in tap water. The minerals such as chlorine and potential toxins, however, are not removed. So you may want to think about using filtered water for recipes that use water you'll be drinking, such as in soups and smoothies.

You could also take it a step further and use filtered water for cooking grains, such as pasta and rice. The small amounts of minerals, chlorine, and potential pollutants absorbed by pasta or rice won't send you to the hospital with lead poisoning. Using tap water sparingly and in combination with bottled and/or filtered water when cooking may be a good way to balance convenience with rigor when it comes to using water in the kitchen.

RECIPES

Breakfast

5-MINUTE MUESLI

3 cups whole oats

3 cups fruit-juice-sweetened cold breakfast cereal*

1 cup dried figs (15 figs), chopped

4 Tbsp flaxseeds, ground or whole

1/2 cup walnuts, chopped

1/4 cup pumpkin seeds

Combine ingredients in a bowl and stir. Serve in a bowl with 1 cup of organic, low-fat milk or unsweetened soymilk. Store the rest in an airtight container for up to 3 months. Makes 8 servings.

Radha McLean

THE TASTE TEST

This super easy recipe makes the perfect breakfast for a pregnant mommy: tasty, hearty, healthy, and easy. The combination of whole grains, nuts, and fruit will keep you chewing this chunky goodness for minutes and fill your belly for hours.

LITTLE LESSON

Make a single or double recipe and store it in a jar or in the freezer. You'll have an effortless breakfast or snack waiting for you day and night!

IF YOU LIKE

If you like other types of nuts or dried fruit, use them. Figs are used here because they're high in calcium and iron. Apricots and raisins are good alternatives to figs since they're high in folic acid. Don't skip out on the flaxseeds since they're a rare source of ALA. Sunflower and pumpkin seeds are excellent sources of iron and have some ALA too. Plus, all nuts are a healthy source of protein!

*Some brands of fruit-juice-sweetened cold breakfast cereal include Arrowhead Mills, Barbara's, Good Morning and Nature's Path. Contact information for these brands can be found in the Resources chapter. These brands have wheat and gluten-free options.

Nutrition rundown

Carbs	Fat	Sugar	ALA	Calcium	Folic Acid
55 g	15 g	23 g	1835 mg	390 mg	97 mcg
Iron	Protein	Cal	Salt	Fiber	
7 mg	22 g	503	207 mg	10 g	

10-MINUTE SCRAMBLED EGG-LESS

1 15-ounce block firm tofu, crumbled

1/2 cup organic low-fat cheddar cheese or vegan
    cheddar cheese, grated

1 cup organic baby spinach

1 Tbsp canola oil

1 medium red onion, peeled and thinly diced

1 cup organic mushrooms, chopped with stems
    removed

1 Tbsp nutritional yeast flakes*

1 Tbsp soy sauce

1 Tbsp fresh or 1 tsp dried thyme or basil

4 small whole grain tortillas

1/4 cup salsa

Place canola oil in a saucepan on medium-high heat. Add
onions. Sauté for 3–4 minutes, or until translucent. Add
tofu. Sauté for another 5 minutes. Add mushrooms and
spinach. Stir, cover, then lower heat to medium-low and
cook for 5 minutes. Uncover, add cheese, nutritional yeast
and soy sauce. Stir, cover, then cook for an additional
5 minutes. Warm tortillas in a toaster oven or oven for
3 minutes at 200 degrees. Place filling on one side of
tortillas, place 2 tablespoons of salsa inside, then fold
tortillas in half. Serve immediately. Makes 4 servings.

THE TASTE TEST

Trick your loved ones into eating this faux greasy, cheesy, gooey mess of a nutritious breakfast. Oozing with protein, vitamins, and healthy ALA, this meal will leave your loved ones—including baby-to-be—licking their chops.

LITTLE LESSONS

Tofu packs a wallop of protein, calcium and fiber. It's a great substitute for eggs in any meal, including pie and cookie recipes.

Flaxseed oil, despite being high in hard-to-find ALA, is not used here because the oil is pan heated. While all types of oil go through oxidation (a chemical reaction that releases toxins) when they are cooked at high temperatures, flaxseed oil produces more of it because of its high ALA content. Canola oil is a good option when pan cooking since it has less ALA than flaxseed oil.

Nutritional yeast flakes are different from the yeast used for baking. This kind of yeast, eaten raw, is high in protein, folic acid, and vitamin B. It can be purchased in containers or in bulk.

LITTLE TIPS

Cheese, soy sauce, and nutritional yeast are all high in sodium, so you do not need to add salt to this recipe.

If you simply love eggs, especially for breakfast, try this recipe with 6 egg whites using free-range organic eggs.

If you're allergic to wheat, serve with corn tortillas, or on top of wheat-free bread.

*Red Star is one brand of nutritional yeast flakes. Contact information for Red Star can be found in the Resources chapter.

Nutrition rundown

Carbs	Fat	Sugar	Omega 3 Fat	Calcium	Folic Acid
33 g	10 g	3 g	673 mg	228 mg	115 mcg

Iron	Protein	Cal	Salt	Fiber
4 mg	20 g	290	619 mg	6 g

MULTIGRAIN COFFEE "CAKE"

1 cup soy flour

1/2 cup whole wheat flour

1/2 cup unbleached white enriched wheat flour

1 cup organic low-fat milk or unsweetened soymilk

1/4 cup unsweetened low-fat organic yogurt or soy yogurt

1/4 cup plus 1 tsp canola oil

1/2 cup maple syrup

1 Tbsp white vinegar

1 Tbsp vanilla

1 Tbsp baking powder

1 tsp cinnamon

1/4 tsp nutmeg

1/4 tsp baking soda

Parchment paper

Preheat oven to 350 degrees F. Grease a 9 x 9 baking pan with 1 teaspoon of oil, then line with parchment paper and set aside.

Place soy, whole wheat, and enriched white flour together in a flour sifter. Sift into a mixing bowl. Place baking powder and soda into the sifter. Sift into the bowl. Add cinnamon and nutmeg. Stir. In a separate bowl, combine soymilk, oil, yogurt, maple syrup, vanilla, and vinegar. Stir. In three batches, add wet ingredients to dry ingredients. Mix together until smooth. Do not over mix. Pour batter into prepared baking pan. Place in oven and bake for approximately 30 minutes, until cake is firm in the middle and does not stick to a toothpick. Remove from oven. Let cool then remove parchment paper from bottom of cake. Makes 8 servings.

THE TASTE TEST

This shockingly delicious "cake" is serious competition for other healthy breakfast options such as cereal, toast, muffin or pastry. This recipe includes soy and whole wheat flour, whole grain flours with more fiber and protein than white (refine wheat) flour. It also uses maple syrup, an unrefined sweetener, and has fewer grams of sugar compared to traditional breakfast muffins and pastries—what more could a hungry pregnant mommy ask for?

LITTLE LESSON

Replace some white flour in any baking recipe with whole wheat and soy flour—they're lower in carbs and higher in ALA, calcium and protein.

IF YOU LIKE

If you like nuts, then add them. Chopped walnuts would add ALA, calcium, and zinc. If you just want the ALA without the nuts, add 1 tablespoon of ground flaxseeds. You'll get the benefits of ALA without even noticing!

Radha McLean

LITTLE TIPS

You can make the flour mix in advance, or double the recipe and store it in the freezer for up to 3 months.

For a wheat-free recipe, use barley or spelt flour instead of wheat flour. For a gluten-free recipe, use gluten-free baking mix instead of wheat flour.

Nutrition rundown

Carbs	Fat	Sugar	ALA	Calcium	Folic Acid
32 g	10 g	14 g	1425 mg	194 mg	45 mcg
Iron	Protein	Cal	Salt	Fiber	
2 mg	7 g	239	246 mg	2 g	

MADE FOR BABY OMEGA OATMEAL

1 cup steel cut oats

2 1/4 cups organic low-fat milk or unsweetened soymilk

2 cups water

1/2 cup organic apple, peeled and finely diced, or
    unsweetened apple sauce

1 Tbsp pure vanilla

1/4 tsp ground cloves

1/4 cup walnuts, chopped

1 Tbsp flaxseeds, ground

Optional: 1 Tbsp honey

Combine water and 2 cups milk in a saucepan. Bring to
a boil. Add oats and apple chunks or sauce. Bring to a
boil, then lower heat to simmer. Add vanilla and cloves.
Cook for approximately 25 minutes on simmer, stirring
frequently. Consistency should be thick and stew like
without sticking to the bottom of pan. Remove from
heat. Add walnuts, flaxseeds, and 1/4 cup milk. If you
want more sweetness, add honey. Stir. Makes 4 servings.

THE TASTE TEST

This warm, hearty, chunky, yet delectably creamy meal
is naturally sweet (the vanilla and cooked fruit infuses
sweetness without adding sugar) and packed with
nutrients (the oats and milk both have lots of calcium
and folic acid) and healthy fat (flaxseeds and walnuts
have hard-to-find ALA) that's great for your baby's brain
development. The hint of cloves gives it a rustic bite that
will leave your baby kicking with satisfaction. Serve for

breakfast or even a snack and you won't even *think* about food for hours afterward!

LITTLE LESSON

Instant and even whole oats are not as fibrous as steel cut oats. Steel cut oats are the original form of the oat and therefore are the highest in fiber and nutritional value of the three forms.

IF YOU LIKE

You can use your favorite dried or fresh fruit instead of apple. Dried or fresh apricots, pears or berries would be equally delicious.

Quick quinoa
For a quicker, high-protein version of this recipe, make it with 3/4 cup quinoa flakes* instead of oatmeal. Add the quinoa flakes to 1 1/2 cups of boiling water. Continue to boil for 20 seconds. Remove from heat, stir with a fork, and cover for another minute. Add cloves, nuts, fruit, and milk or milk substitute, and stir.

---

*One brand of quinoa flakes is Ancient Harvest. Contact information for Ancient Harvest can be found in the Resources chapter.

Nutrition rundown

Carbs	Fat	Sugar	ALA	Calcium	Folic Acid
41g	10g	14g	1.1 g	199 mg	38 mcg
Iron	Protein	Cal	Salt	Fiber	
2 mg	13 g	302	63 mg	6 g	

COFFEE CRAVERS' CREATION

3/4 cup instant grain-based beverage*

3/4 cup organic low-fat milk or unsweetened soy milk

2 Tbsp unsweetened cocoa powder

2 Tbsp maple syrup

2 Tbsp unsweetened chocolate or plain protein powder

2 cups ice cubes

Boil 3/4 cup of water. Place powered grain-based beverage (amount of powder as indicated on container) and cocoa powder in a cup. Add hot water. Mix until both powders are dissolved. Place warm drink, maple syrup, protein powder, and ice cubes in a blender. Puree until smooth. Makes 2 servings.

THE TASTE TEST

This drink is the perfect fix for coffee addicts resisting that daily cup while baby is on board, and for anyone who loves iced drinks or smoothies. You'll suck up this made-for-pregnancy drink almost as quickly as it took to make it. The instant beverage mix made from whole grains (barley, chicory, and rye), tastes uncannily similar to coffee without the caffeine. Plus, the use of maple syrup instead of white (refined cane) sugar and added protein powder make this pregnancy-friendly creation higher in protein than store-bought coffee drinks without the refined sugar.

LITTLE LESSON

Caffeinated coffee is not good to consume during your pregnancy since it contains a lot of caffeine, a stimulant that increases your blood pressure and is transferred to your baby. Caffeine is also a diuretic that makes you lose water. Try drinking decaf and making drinks such as this one with an all-natural, grain-based beverage, which has a rich, hearty taste that mimics the flavor of coffee.

*One brand of instant grain-based beverage is Pero. Contact information for Pero can be found in the Resources chapter.

Nutrition rundown

Carbs	Fat	Sugar	Omega 3 Fat	Calcium	Folic Acid
24 g	2 g	15 g	35 mg	316 mg	25 mcg
Iron	Protein	Cal	Salt	Fiber	
6 mg	10 g	144	118 mg	2 g	

BLUEBERRY BUZZ

1 1/2 cups organic blueberries, frozen

1 cup organic low-fat milk or unsweetened soymilk

1 cup ice cubes

1/2 cup filtered water

1/4 cup organic unsweetened apple sauce

2 Tbsp unsweetened chocolate protein powder

Place wet ingredients in blender first, then add dry ingredients. Puree until smooth. Makes 4 servings.

THE TASTE TEST

This quick fix drink is high in protein and low in carbs—without an empty carb in sight. The fruit/apple sauce combo makes it super sweet without the need for processed sugars or even juice. The milk and protein powder pack in the protein and add the creamy consistency of a milkshake without the fat and processed sugar in ice cream. This shake is a great bedtime or afternoon snack that will make you forget about that urge for ice cream or cake (or both).

LITTLE LESSON

Replace juice with whole fruit whenever possible. Many protein shakes, including those sold in stores, are made with fruit juice, which is high in sugar without the benefits of fiber. Not to mention the fact that many brands of fruit juice are made with added refined sugar. Adding unsweetened apple sauce or frozen, chopped fruit to smoothies instead of juice gives the same juicy flavor without the empty carbs of juice itself.

IF YOU LIKE

If you like another type of fruit, use it instead. Organic berries, in particular, are highly recommended because the conventionally grown versions are covered with pesticides. If you cannot find organic berries or organic fruit in general, opt for conventionally grown bananas, pears, plums, kiwis, mangos or other fruit with peels that can be removed.

Nutrition rundown

Carbs	Fat	Sugar	ALA	Calcium	Folic Acid
31 g	3 g	23 g	194 mg	626 mg	60 mcg
Iron	Protein	Cal	Salt	Fiber	
12 mg	20 g	227	230 mg	4 g	

HUNGER-STOPPING HUMMUS

1 15-ounce can garbanzo beans

1/4 cup liquid from can beans

1/4 cup tahini

1 Tbsp plus 1 tsp lemon juice

1 Tbsp flaxseed oil

1 clove garlic, peeled and crushed

1/2 tsp salt

1/4 tsp pepper

Place wet ingredients in a food processor or blender first, then add dry ingredients. Puree until smooth. Makes 6 servings. Eat with your favorite raw veggies such as carrots or celery, or with whole wheat pita bread if you're extra hungry between meals.

THE TASTE TEST

This super filling creamy-oily spread makes for a hearty between-meal snack. High in fiber, protein, and healthy fats, it will surely cure that craving for junk food and sweets—at least until your baby starts kicking for his or her next meal.

LITTLE LESSONS

The tahini and beans have plenty of protein, fiber, and ALA, and the flaxseed oil packs in the ALA fat with 7 grams in a tablespoon. Add even as little as 1 teaspoon of flaxseed oil to any snack dip, spread or salad dressing to get your fill of ALA for the day (1.4 grams a day).

If you like

If you prefer to exclude flaxseed oil, use canola or walnut oil instead—both are high in ALA as well but have milder flavors than flaxseed oil.

Nutrition rundown

Carbs	Fat	Sugar	ALA	Calcium	Folic Acid
17 g	9 g	3 g	1.3 g	39 mg	57 mcg
Iron	Protein	Cal	Salt	Fiber	
2 mg	6 g	168	315 mg	5 g	

SIMPLY HEALTHY SORBET CUPS

2 cups organic low-fat milk or unsweetened soymilk

1 cup organic strawberries or other berries, frozen

2 organic bananas, frozen and sliced

4 empty 6-ounce yogurt containers with lids, cleaned and dried

Place milk in the blender first, then add frozen fruit. Puree until smooth, stopping blender and mixing ingredients well if blades of the blender get stuck. Pour into 4 yogurt containers evenly. Place lids on top of containers. Place them on an even surface in the freezer. Freeze for at least one hour (you can keep them in the freezer for up to 3 months). When ready to eat, remove from freezer and thaw at room temperature for 10 minutes or heat in the microwave for 15–20 seconds. Makes 4 servings.

THE TASTE TEST

These refreshing and tasty cups made of pure fruit and milk are the perfect alternative to ice cream, frozen yogurt or store-bought sorbet, most of which are made with refined sugar, artificial sweeteners, chemical additives and/or preservatives.

LITTLE LESSON

This sorbet has nutrients a pregnant mommy needs, with protein and iron in the milk and fruit and folic acid in the soymilk (if used). So if you're craving more after having one, go ahead—eat two!

Nutrition rundown

Carbs	Fat	Sugar	ALA	Calcium	Folic Acid
24 g	3 g	16 g	0 mg	155 mg	27 mcg

Iron	Protein	Cal	Salt	Fiber
1 mg	5 g	133	51 mg	3 g

Wow! It's WHEAT-FREE BANANA BREAD

1 cup barley flour

1/2 cup plus 1 tsp oat flour

1/2 cup plus 1 tsp canola oil

2 extra-ripe organic bananas, mashed

3/4 cup maple syrup

1/2 cup walnuts, chopped

1/3 cup organic low-fat sour cream, unsweetened yogurt
   or soy yogurt

1 Tbsp lecithin soaked in 2 Tbsp warm water

1 tsp baking powder

1/4 tsp salt

Preheat oven to 350 degrees F. Grease and flour an 8-inch square pan with 1 teaspoon of canola oil and 1 teaspoon of oat flour. In a medium-sized mixing bowl, stir sour cream or yogurt and maple syrup together. Add bananas and lecithin. Sift the flours and baking powder through a flour sifter and mix together in a separate bowl. Blend the wet ingredients into the dry ingredients. Add chopped nuts. Stir well. Pour into the baking pan and bake for 25–30 minutes, until cake is firm in the middle and does not stick to a toothpick. Makes 12 servings.

THE TASTE TEST

This scrumptious, moist bread is the perfect whole grain treat for those allergic to wheat. The allergy-prone and wheat lovers alike will enjoy the glorious combination of fluffy cake, naturally sweet bananas, creamy yogurt, and crunchy nuts for an evening or midnight snack—maybe even enough to keep you sleeping all night long.

LITTLE LESSONS

Barley flour is whole grain flour that has more protein, calcium, fiber, and ALA than white (refined wheat) flour and more calcium and ALA than whole wheat flour. So it's an excellent choice for baking regardless of whether or not you're allergic to wheat (it is not gluten-free). Since barley flour is dense, however, be sure to combine it with oat flour, which is lighter and fluffier when baked. Plus, oat flour contains some calcium, folic acid, and protein, too.

Lecithin is an emulsifier made from soy oil that acts like eggs to help the ingredients in cakes bind together. Lecithin is a good alternative to eggs to use in baking.

LITTLE TIPS

For a gluten-free recipe, use 1 1/2 cups of gluten-free baking mix instead of barley and oat flour.

Whole grain baking mix, now sold in supermarkets and online, is a convenient and healthy way to bake cakes, cookies and quick breads without having to mix the different flours together from scratch.

Nutrition rundown

Carbs	Fat	Sugar	ALA	Calcium	Folic Acid
22 g	14 g	10 g	1.1 g	80 mg	37 mcg
Iron	Protein	Cal	Salt	Fiber	
1 mg	4 g	217	128 mg	2 g	

Amazing ALA salad

Salad ingredients

4 cups organic baby spinach

1 cup organic white button mushrooms, cut into quarters with stems removed

1/2 cup part-skim fresh mozzarella cheese (organic if you can find it), cut into 1/2 inch chunks

1 cup organic cherry tomatoes, cut into halves

1 mango, peeled, pitted, and cut into small chunks

1/4 cup whole walnuts

1 Tbsp sunflower seeds

Dressing ingredients

2 Tbsp organic unsweetened low-fat yogurt or soy
   yogurt

1 Tbsp flaxseed oil

1 Tbsp olive oil

1 Tbsp honey mustard

1 Tbsp white vinegar

1 Tbsp lime juice

1 Tbsp fresh oregano or dried oregano

1/2 tsp salt

1/4 tsp pepper

Combine all salad ingredients in a large mixing bowl.
Place dressing ingredients in a bowl. Beat vigorously with
a mixer or fork until it emulsifies (becomes creamy). Pour
over salad and mix well. Makes 4 servings.

THE TASTE TEST

You will be floored by the fabulous flavors in this
decadent, deceptively healthy salad. The exotic flavor of
the mango smothered in the creamy, tangy dressing will
leave you hallucinating about palm trees and azure seas.
Add the crunch of the nuts and fresh vegetables, and
you'll feel as if you ate a savory meal and sweet dessert
all in one.

LITTLE LESSONS

ALA is the centerpiece of this dish, with 2.7 grams in a
serving. Walnuts and flaxseed oil are both high in this
omega fat that's needed for your baby's brain development.

Throw either of these toppings on any salad or stir fry and you'll get your (and baby's) fill of much-needed ALA for the day.

The spinach and sunflower seeds are also excellent ingredients to use in salad since they have iron, folic acid and protein. Plus, the mango and tomatoes are high in vitamin C, so they help your body absorb all that iron.

IF YOU LIKE

If you like a less creamy dressing, use water instead of yogurt. Also, you can replace mango with apple, papaya, kiwi, peach, nectarine, pear or plum in the salad if you can't find, don't like or are allergic to mango. If you don't like the taste of flaxseed oil, use canola oil instead.

Nutrition rundown

Carbs	Fat	Sugar	ALA	Calcium	Folic Acid
22 g	20 g	10 g	2.7 g	295 mg	131 mcg

Iron	Protein	Cal	Salt	Fiber
2 mg	13 g	350	519 mg	8g

Eco-friendly kale quesadillas

8 small whole grain tortillas

1 cup organic low-fat cheese or vegan cheese, grated

1 organic avocado, pitted and cut into half-inch chunks

1 head organic kale, chopped with stems removed

1 medium organic onion, peeled and chopped

1/4 cup salsa

2 Tbsp cold water

1 Tbsp canola oil

1 Tbsp lemon juice

1 Tbsp Bragg Liquid Aminos*

1/8 tsp pepper

Cooking spray

Optional: 1/4 cup pineapple, cut into small chunks

To make the kale

Place canola oil in a saucepan over high heat. Let oil heat in pan for 1 minute. Add onion. Sauté onions for 3-4 minutes, until translucent. Add kale. Coat kale with onions and oil by turning the kale over several times. Add lemon juice, Bragg Liquid Aminos and water. Lower heat to simmer, cover and let cook for 10 minutes, stirring frequently. Taste kale to make sure veins are tender and well cooked. Remove from heat.

To make the salsa

Combine the salsa, avocado, and pineapple chunks (if using them) in a bowl and mix. Set aside.

To make the quesadillas

Place a stainless steel or cast-iron saucepan over low-medium heat. Spray cooking oil on the surface. Place one tortilla in saucepan. Sprinkle 1/4 of cheese and kale/onion sauté evenly across top. Place second tortilla on top of ingredients. Cook for 2 minutes, until bottom tortilla begins to crisp. Flip quesadillas over carefully using a spatula. Cook other side for 2 minutes, until bottom tortilla begins to crisp. Check inside to make sure that cheese is melted. Remove from pan and place on a plate.

Repeat this process until you've made 4 quesadillas. If you are not serving immediately, place on a baking sheet in the oven at 200 degrees a few minutes before serving. When ready to serve, place a single quesadilla on a plate. Sprinkle salsa on top. Slice into quarters. Eat with abandon. Makes 4 servings.

THE TASTE TEST

These quesadillas, which play off the traditional Mexican version made with conventional (non-organic) cheese or beef alone, surpass the real thing in eco-friendliness and nutritional value with flying colors. The lack of meat and use of whole grain tortillas, organic kale, and organic low-fat cheese minimize the toxins, empty carbs and negative impact on the environment while packing in the vitamins, minerals, and fiber. But don't be fooled by the green and healthy ingredient; you'll inhale the tasty cheese, avocado, and salsa, which disguise all of those vitamins pretty darn well.

LITTLE LESSON

Kale is among the most nutritious of all vegetables, with lots of calcium, folic acid, fiber, and iron. It takes a few minutes longer to prepare and is harder to cook than spinach or broccoli since its veins and leaves are generally tough and bitter before cooking. This recipe is a tried-and-true favorite for a mouth-watering meal with kale you'll barely notice.

IF YOU LIKE

If you like sour cream on your quesadillas, use low-fat organic sour cream, unsweetened yogurt or soy sour cream.

If you miss the ground beef, try adding 1/4 cup of textured vegetable protein soaked in water to the kale once it is cooked. If you don't like the taste of flaxseed oil, use canola oil instead.

LITTLE TIPS

Bragg Liquid Aminos is an excellent replacement for salt or soy sauce. Made from soy beans, this salty-tasting dressing is lower in sodium than table salt and soy sauce.

If you're allergic to wheat, use corn tortillas instead of whole grain tortillas.

If you use vegan cheese, some brands don't melt well, so test out different brands to find one that melts to your liking.

*Contact information for Bragg Liquid Aminos can be found in the Resources chapter.

Nutrition rundown

Carbs	Fat	Sugar	ALA	Calcium	Folic Acid
53 g	13 g	3 g	734 mg	152 mg	81 mcg
Iron	Protein	Cal	Salt	Fiber	
3 mg	17 g	380	734 mg	9 g	

FABULOUS FOUR BEAN SALAD

Salad ingredients

1 15-ounce can black beans

1 15-ounce can kidney beans

1 15-ounce can cannellini beans

1 15-ounce can garbanzo beans

2 sticks organic celery, finely diced with the ends removed

2 organic plum tomatoes, finely diced

1 large organic carrot, peeled and finely diced

1 small organic red onion, peeled and finely diced

Dressing ingredients

3 Tbsp olive oil

1 Tbsp flaxseed oil

1 Tbsp honey mustard

1 Tbsp white vinegar

1 Tbsp lime juice

1 Tbsp fresh oregano or 1 tsp dried oregano

1/2 tsp salt

1/4 tsp pepper

Combine all salad ingredients in a large bowl and mix. Combine dressing ingredients in a bowl and beat vigorously with a mixer or fork until it emulsifies (becomes creamy). Add dressing to salad and mix. Makes 6 servings.

THE TASTE TEST

This incredibly easy-to-make bean salad tastes like anything but instant. The array of beans and acids in the dressing makes for a quick, fabulous tasting and unexpectedly filling meal.

LITTLE LESSONS

Foods high in protein and fiber fill you up for longer periods of time because your body takes more time to process nutrients compared to foods with less protein and/or fiber. High protein foods also keep your blood sugar "even" by avoiding peaks in blood sugar. Foods with less protein cause your body to produce more insulin, making your blood sugar peak then drop, thus leading you to feel hungry sooner after eating.

This meal is also high in ALA—1.4 grams a serving. Aside from the flaxseed oil in the dressing (a great way to add ALA to your daily meals), white, black, and kidney beans have notable amounts of ALA as well.

IF YOU LIKE

If you like other types of beans, such as black-eyed peas, lentils, lima beans or peas, or different vegetables such as cucumbers or peppers, feel free to use them instead. Making your food as tasty as possible by using your favorite foods is the key to eating healthfully while also satisfying your hunger.

Nutrition rundown

Carbs	Fat	Sugar	ALA	Calcium	Folic Acid
48 g	13 g	4 g	1.4 g	110 mg	172 mcg

Iron	Protein	Cal	Salt	Fiber
5 mg	14 g	336	649 mg	14 g

WHOLE GRAIN DINNER CREPES WITH CHEESE-ASPARAGUS-WALNUT FILLING

Crepe ingredients

1 1/2 cup buckwheat flour

1/2 cup soy flour

1 1/4 cup organic low-fat milk or unsweetened soymilk

1 1/4 cup filtered water

1 Tbsp butter or margarine, melted

1/2 tsp salt

Filling ingredients

2 cups organic low-fat cheese or vegan cheese, grated

1 organic shallot or white onion, peeled and finely chopped

1 cup organic asparagus, cut into 2-inch pieces with ends removed

1/2 cup walnuts, finely chopped

1 Tbsp butter or margarine, melted

Salt and pepper

Cooking spray

To make the batter

Place two types of flour in a flour sifter and sift into a medium-sized mixing bowl. Add salt and mix. Place milk and water in a small bowl and mix well. Stir wet ingredients into the flour in 3 batches, stirring until smooth. Cover bowl with a cloth napkin and refrigerate for one hour or overnight.

To make the filling

Place cooking spray and 1 tablespoon of butter in a hot sauté pan. Let butter melt. Add diced shallots or onion, sprinkle with a pinch of salt and pepper, and stir frequently for 2 minutes.

Wash and pat dry asparagus. Cut off the ends (by about 2 inches). Slice thinly at 45 degree angle so that pieces look like small arrows. Add asparagus and walnuts to shallots. Lower heat to low-medium, cover and cook for 10 minutes, stirring occasionally. Grate cheese and set aside. When filling is done cooking, place in a bowl next to a sauté pan you'll use to make the crepes. (Crepes cook quickly, so keeping all your utensils and ingredients within reach makes the cooking process easier).

To make the crepes

When batter has been cooled, remove from refrigerator and place next to the pan. Place a stainless steel or cast-iron pan on high heat. Spray with cooking spray. Heat for 2 minutes. Lower heat to medium.

Using a soup ladle, scoop approximately three-fourths cup of batter onto the middle of the pan. Place the bottom of ladle gently on top of the batter and spread the batter in a circular motion. Cook for 1–2 minutes, until edges are firm and bubbles are popped. Using a spatula, gently flip crepe over. Place cheese and asparagus filling on half of pancake and fold one side without the filling across the top. Cook for 1 minute, then flip over. Cook another minute, then remove from pan and place on a cookie sheet (you can easily reheat crepes if placed directly on a cookie sheet). Repeat this process until you've made 6 crepes. Makes 6 servings.

THE TASTE TEST

This wholesome take on a crepe is the closest thing you'll get to the real thing during your pregnancy without the empty carbs. Traditional crepes, made with whole eggs and a lot of butter and white (refined wheat) flour, are far from nutritious. But you'll gobble down this homemade version designed just for a pregnant woman. The buckwheat and soy flour add a nutty, hearty flavor that's equally flavorful and much more filling (you'll be done eating for hours after having one of these). The cheese-walnut-asparagus filling does not disappoint the taste buds either, with equal richness as a traditional dinner crepe.

LITTLE LESSONS

Buckwheat is an incredibly filling whole grain. Why? Because it's higher in protein, fiber, iron, and folic acid than refined wheat flour. Asparagus has one of the highest amounts of folic acid of all vegetables, so it's a great choice for any dinner recipe.

Walnuts are used here because they've got ALA, plus protein and fiber to boot.

Nutrition rundown

Carbs	Fat	Sugar	ALA	Calcium	Folic Acid
29 g	14 g	5 g	1.1 g	438 mg	67 mcg
Iron	Protein	Cal	Salt	Fiber	
3 mg	20 g	322	324 mg	5 g	

Hearty kasha and veggies

3 cups water

1 cup roasted buckwheat (brown)

1 Tbsp powdered or 1 cube mock chicken or vegetable broth

1 Tbsp plus 1 tsp olive oil

2 medium organic carrots, peeled and thinly sliced

1 medium organic onion, peeled and finely chopped

1 organic zucchini, sliced with the ends removed

1 Tbsp sesame seeds

1 Tbsp Bragg Liquid Aminos*

2 tsp cumin

1/2 tsp plus one pinch of salt

Place a large stainless steel or cast-iron pan over medium heat. Add 1 teaspoon of olive oil and one pinch of salt. Place buckwheat in the pan and roast for 5 minutes, stirring frequently to prevent burning. In a separate saucepan, bring 2 1/2 cups of water to a boil. Add vegetable broth to boiling water. Add boiling water to kasha and reduce heat to low-medium. Cover and cook until all the water is absorbed, approximately 25–30 minutes.

Place medium pan over medium-high heat. Add 1 tablespoon of olive oil and onions. Sauté for 3-4 minutes, until translucent. Add carrots, cumin and 1/2 cup water. Reduce heat, cover and cook for 5 minutes. Stir frequently. Add zucchini and 1/2 tsp salt. Cook for 3–4 minutes, until zucchini is tender. Place sautéed vegetables over cooked kasha. Top with sesame seeds and Bragg Liquid Aminos. Makes 4 servings.

THE TASTE TEST

This hearty meal of warm, roasted whole grains and delicately cooked vegetables makes for a filling, nutritious dinner. The buckwheat, or kasha, is packed with protein, fiber, and B vitamins so you'll be sure to fill up your and baby's belly until dawn.

LITTLE LESSON

Kasha is the Polish or Russian name for buckwheat, the high fiber and protein grain used in the crepe recipes in this book. This grain has been a staple of Eastern European cuisine for centuries and for good reason: It is a complete protein that contains all the protein, complex carbs, and amino acids (molecules that are the building blocks of protein) you need in one meal.

*Contact information for Bragg Liquid Aminos can be found in the Resources chapter.

Nutrition rundown

Carbs	Fat	Sugar	Omega 3 Fat	Calcium	Folic Acid
27 g	7 g	4 g	65 mg	48 mg	37 mcg

Iron	Protein	Cal	Salt	Fiber
2 mg	15 g	175	502 mg	5 g

In-a-minute minestrone soup

This soup uses the Fabulous four bean salad recipe on page 79 in this book. Simply add your bean salad leftovers to this dish to make a delicious new meal in minutes.

2 servings Fabulous four bean salad

6 cups filtered water

2 cups tomato puree

1 cup whole wheat elbow noodles

Combine water and tomato puree in a medium-sized pot over high heat. Bring to a boil. Add leftover four bean salad and elbow noodles. Bring to a boil again, then lower heat to low, cover and cook for 10 minutes. Makes 4 servings.

The taste test

This soup is convenient for pregnant moms who are too busy or tired (or both) to cook a new recipe for every meal. This soup has the same benefits as the four bean salad—high in fiber, iron, and protein—yet tastes like a new meal altogether.

Little lesson

When cooking with water that you will actually drink (for example, in soups) use filtered water if possible. While you may think that tap water is clean, most tap water contains trace amounts of numerous potentially harmful items including bacteria, chlorine, pesticides, rust, and even pharmaceutical medications.

LITTLE TIP

Use corn, quinoa, rice or any other type of gluten-free elbow noodles instead of whole wheat noodles if you're allergic to wheat or gluten.

Nutrition rundown

Carbs	Fat	Sugar	ALA	Calcium	Folic Acid
55 g	7 g	8 g	716 mg	88 mg	115 mcg
Iron	Protein	Cal	Salt	Fiber	
6 mg	13 g	307	357 mg	12 g	

RED 'N "GREEN" PIZZA

4 pieces large whole grain pita or flat bread

1 cup organic low-fat mozzarella cheese or vegan cheese, grated

2 large organic beefsteak tomatoes, cut into fourths

2 packed cups organic baby spinach

2 cloves organic garlic, peeled and finely chopped

1 Tbsp canola oil

1 Tbsp organic fresh or 1 tsp dried oregano

1/4 tsp pepper

Preheat oven to broil. Place spinach in a food processor or blender. Using the pulse function, cut until spinach is very finely chopped. (Be sure not to chop too long. If you do, it will become pureed.) Scoop spinach out of food processor and place in a bowl.

Place tomatoes, spinach, oregano, garlic, and pepper in the food processor or blender. Pulse until very finely chopped. Scoop out and place in the bowl with the spinach. Mix well. Pour mixture into a strainer with a bowl underneath. Strain the excess water from the sauce by stirring and patting the sauce gently. Place back into a bowl.

On a baking sheet, place pitas or pieces of flat bread evenly. Place in the oven on a rack positioned in the middle vertically, not too close to the top burners. Broil for 2 minutes, or until bread turns a light, crispy brown. Remove from oven. Turn bread over so that the cooked sides are face down. Brush tops with canola oil. Place back into the oven and broil for 2 minutes, or until bread turns a light, crispy brown. Remove from oven.

With a spoon, scoop sauce and place evenly on top of each piece of bread. Sprinkle cheese evenly on top of each piece. Place in the oven and broil for 3-4 minutes, until cheese is melted and browned. Remove from oven. Cool for a few minutes then slice each piece into fourths. Serve immediately and eat to your heart's content! Makes 4 servings.

THE TASTE TEST

This organic recipe is a fantastic alternative to store- or restaurant-bought pizza. The whole grain pita or flatbread makes for a more filling and nutritious crust since it has more folic acid, iron, ALA, and protein than regular pizza crust made from white (refined wheat) flour. The red 'n "green" sauce made with organic tomatoes, spinach, herbs and spices disguises the missing traditional pizza dough and full-fat cheese by packing in a punch of delicious flavors.

LITTLE LESSON

The bread, cheese, spinach, and tomato combo in pizza is an excellent way to get iron: The bread, cheese and spinach have iron while tomatoes have lots of vitamin C, which helps your body absorb all that iron.

IF YOU LIKE

If you like pizza, make it yourself using whole grain bread and organic low-fat cheese. You'll enjoy the gooey goodness without the empty carbs of refined wheat flour and the soaring fat content of regular cheese.

LITTLE TIPS

Don't add extra salt to your pizza—bread, cheese, and premade tomato sauce are all high in salt.

Piling your dishes high with chopped vegetables and herbs eliminates the need for high fat, processed and salty ingredients. Add your favorite vegetables, herbs, and spices in place of oils, fried food, meats and empty carbs to a meal and you'll create an unbeatable symphony of flavors every time!

Use gluten-free bread or corn tortillas instead of whole grain pita bread or flatbread if you're allergic to wheat or gluten.

Nutrition rundown

Carbs	Fat	Sugar	ALA	Calcium	Folic Acid
42 g	10 g	3 g	754 mg	265 mg	72 mcg
Iron	Protein	Cal	Salt	Fiber	
3 mg	16 g	307	507 mg	7 g	

ROASTED VEGGIE BLOWOUT

3 cups water

1 cup quinoa

1 large organic carrot, peeled and thinly sliced

1 cup organic mushrooms, cut into fourths with the stems removed

1 cup organic cauliflower, cut into large chunks with the core removed

1 cup organic brussel sprouts, cut into fourths with the stems removed

1 15-ounces block tofu, cut into 1-inch chunks

1 medium onion, peeled and thinly sliced

2 Tbsp canola oil

1 Tbsp fresh or 1 tsp dried thyme

1 Tbsp soy sauce

1/2 tsp salt

1/4 tsp white pepper

To make the quinoa

Place 1 cup quinoa and 3 cups water in a stainless steel rice cooker.* Turn it on. Set aside. (It will cook on its own in 30 minutes.) If you don't have a rice cooker, place quinoa and water in a pot over high heat. Bring to a boil. Lower heat to medium-low, cover and let cook for 25-30 minutes.

Radha McLean

To make the vegetables

Preheat oven to broil. Put tofu and prepared vegetables into a large mixing bowl. Add oil and spices. Mix until tofu and vegetables are coated with the oil and spices.

Spread onto a large baking sheet. Place in oven with oven rack close to the bottom of oven. Broil for 10 minutes. Turn ingredients over using a wooden mixing spoon. Cook for another 10 minutes, watching to avoid (black) charring of the vegetables. Remove from oven. Let cool for 10 minutes. Serve over 1/2 cup of cooked quinoa. Makes 4 servings.

THE TASTE TEST

In half an hour, you'll prepare a divine dinner that will leave both mommy and baby sighing with satisfaction. The roasting process releases the natural juices of the vegetables, making them explode with flavor.

LITTLE LESSONS

Quinoa is an exceptionally nutritious grain high in fiber, iron, and protein.

If you do not have a stainless steel rice cooker, consider buying one.* (Many rice cookers are made with aluminum, which can leach toxic aluminum into your food, so a stainless steel rice cooker is the way to go). They're inexpensive and provide a low-maintenance way to cook grains. By the time you're done chopping and cooking the roasted vegetables, the quinoa will be done cooking.

IF YOU LIKE

If you don't like quinoa or cannot find it at your grocery store, replace quinoa with brown rice or whole wheat couscous. Brown rice is crunchier than quinoa, and couscous is more convenient to make. Cook brown rice in a rice cooker or pot following the same instructions as the quinoa (1 cup of rice to 3 cups of water). To cook couscous, place 1 cup couscous into a pot of 2 cups of boiling water. Turn off the heat and stir. Cover and let sit for 10 minutes.

*Contact information for a brand of stainless steel rice cookers can be found in the Resources chapter.

Nutrition rundown

Carbs	Fat	Sugar	ALA	Calcium	Folic Acid
53 g	17 g	4 g	1.3 g	149 mg	123 mcg
Iron	Protein	Cal	Salt	Fiber	
7 mg	22 g	438	596 mg	10 g	

Soy 'n soba noodle soup

8 cups filtered water

1/2 lb soba noodles

1 8-ounce package tofu noodles*

2 packages miso soup mix

1 large organic carrot, peeled and thinly sliced

2 cups organic bok choy or broccoli, cut into 2-inch
pieces with stem removed

1 cup frozen edamame (soybeans), without the pods

1 8-ounce can sliced water chestnuts

1/4 cup dried arame or wakame seaweed, soaked in 1
cup water

2 Tbsp sesame oil

1 Tbsp sesame seeds, roasted

1 tsp dried red pepper flakes

Place 7 cups water in a large saucepan over high heat.
Bring to a boil. Add soba noodles, carrots, edamame, and
bok choy or broccoli. Bring to a boil, then lower heat
to medium and cook for 5 minutes. Add soy noodles,
water chestnuts and seaweed. Cook for an additional 3
minutes. Turn off heat.

Place powered miso soup mix in a medium-sized bowl.
Add 1 cup hot water. Mix with a fork until soup mix
is dissolved. Add dissolved miso soup mix into pot of
noodles and vegetables. To roast sesame seeds, place seeds
in a dry (unoiled) frying pan and cook over medium
heat, stirring continually, for 1 minute. Add sesame oil,
sesame seeds, and red pepper flakes to soup. Stir. Serve in
large soup bowls. Slurp and enjoy! Makes 4 servings.

THE TASTE TEST

The soothing soup is nothing less than a wholesome, filling meal with an array of textures and flavors. The two types of noodles, chunks of vegetables, and silky smooth seaweed will make you feel as if you've eaten for an hour by the time you finish sipping up the broth.

LITTLE LESSONS

Soba noodles are made with whole wheat and buckwheat, the whole grain used in the crepe and kasha recipes, which is higher in fiber and protein than white (refined) wheat or rice noodles. These noodles, which have a nuttier flavor than all-wheat or rice noodles, make a hearty addition to soups and stir fries.

Soy noodles are also a great addition to any soup or stir fry; they are virtually carb free and have some calcium and iron.

Seaweed is a quick-fix way of getting your daily intake of minerals since it's packed with them—seaweed is high in calcium, magnesium, potassium, iodine, iron, and zinc and has smaller amounts of many other trace minerals.

Miso, or fermented soybean paste, is incredibly nutritious. It's high in essential amino acids, vitamin B_{12} and trace minerals such as zinc and copper. A quick note about preparing miso: Don't boil it (boiling miso kills the fermenting fungus that gives miso its healthy properties). Dissolve it in warm water and add it to food after the food has been cooked.

*One brand of tofu noodles is House Foods Tofu Shirataki. Contact information for House Foods Tofu Shirataki can be found in the Resources chapter.

Nutrition rundown

Carbs	Fat	Sugar	ALA	Calcium	Folic Acid
61 g	12 g	3 g	381 mg	158 mg	202 mcg
Iron	Protein	Cal	Salt	Fiber	
4 mg	18 g	394	500 mg	5 g	

BRUNETTE BOMBSHELL PARTY BALLS

1 cup soy nut butter (smooth)*

1/2 cup honey

1/4 cup walnuts, finely chopped

3 Tbsp ground flaxseeds

1 Tbsp soy flour

Candy wrappers or plastic wrap**

Colored twist ties or ribbon, cut into 2-inch pieces**

Parchment paper

Wash and dry hands well. Place soy nut butter and honey in a stainless steel bowl. Fill a double boiler halfway with water and bring water to a boil. Place bowl with nut butter and honey on top of the boiler. With a whisk or mixing spoon, stir continually until they are softened and well mixed. Add soy flour through a flour sifter. Mix well. Remove immediately from heat and let sit for 5 minutes.

Place walnuts and flaxseeds in a coffee grinder, blender or food processor. Chop until the mix becomes powdery. Spread walnut/flaxseed mix on a plate. While soy nut butter/honey mixture is warm, scoop a heaping teaspoon onto a spoon, then roll into individual balls approximately 1 1/2 inches wide using the palms of your hands. Place each ball onto the plate of powdered walnut/flaxseed mix and roll across the plate in a circular motion until the ball is covered with the powder.

Place each ball onto a plate or platter covered with parchment paper. Cover with a cloth napkin and refrigerate for 1 hour. Once the balls are cooled, place them into individual candy wrappers or pieces of plastic wrap and tie colorful twist ties or ribbons on the top. Place the wrapped balls into an air-tight container. The balls can be refrigerated for 1 week or frozen for up to 3 months. Makes 10 servings. Serving size: one ball.

THE TASTE TEST

These high protein "brunette"-colored balls are a perfect snack for any time of day or night—the rich-sweet taste of the soy butter and honey is the closest thing you'll get to a chocolate truffle or candy bar without refined sugar. Plan a "pregnant and healthy" party with your pregnant friends and give these out on a platter or in a gift bag— they'll love the healthy and sweet protein punch of the nut butter/honey combination.

LITTLE LESSONS

Soy nut butter is used because it's higher in calcium and iron than peanut butter (both have folic acid and protein).

Flaxseeds and walnuts, as you may know by now, are a goldmine and rare food source of ALA. So pack the nuts and seeds onto the outsides of these protein powerhouse treats!

Honey is not only a completely natural, chemical-free sweetener, it is known to fight toxic free radicals in the body and has been used as a natural form of medicine for centuries.

LITTLE TIP

If you cannot find soy nut butter, use peanut butter instead. If you're allergic to peanuts, almond butter, and sunflower seed butter are tasty alternatives. If you're allergic to all nuts, soy nut butter is the way to go—just skip the walnuts in the coating.

*One brand of soy nut butter is I.M. Healthy. Contact information for I.M. Healthy soy nut butter can be found in the Resources chapter.

** The Custom Chocolate Shop online sells clear bags (size 2-1/2 x 4-1/4 inches) that you can use as wrappers, and colored metallic twist ties to tie the top of the wrappers. Contact information for The Custom Chocolate Shop can be found in the Resources chapter.

Nutrition rundown

Carbs	Fat	Sugar	ALA	Calcium	Folic Acid
29 g	15 g	21 g	938 mg	142 mg	8 mcg

Iron	Protein	Cal	Salt	Fiber	
0 mg	8 g	276	142 mg	4 g	

"GREEN" LIME PIE

Filling ingredients

3 medium organic avocados (4 cups), peeled and pitted

3/4 cup maple syrup

1/4 cup lime juice

1 large organic banana, peeled and sliced

1 tsp vanilla extract

Crust ingredients

1 1/2 cups almonds

1 1/2 cups coconut, shredded

10 organic medjool dates

1/2 tsp sea salt

Blend avocado, maple syrup, banana, vanilla, and lime juice in a blender or food processor. Set aside. Next, blend almonds, coconut, dates, and sea salt in a food processor until almonds are finely chopped. Press crust mixture into an 8 x 8 x 2 glass baking dish. Pour filling into dish and freeze for 3–4 hours. Remove from the freezer and serve immediately. Keep refrigerated. Makes 10 servings.

THE TASTE TEST

You'll surprise yourself, family and friends by the gourmet quality of this totally green spin on key lime pie—literally and figuratively. The avocado gives the pie its green color, and the recipe is raw and vegan, so it uses environmentally-friendly ingredients and takes almost no energy to make. Offer this healthy treat and at your next dinner party and you'll end up sharing the recipe with everyone!

LITTLE LESSONS

Avocado is rich is glutathione, a potent antioxidant that helps remove toxins from the liver.

This raw, vegan version is full of enzymes (molecules that, among other things, help your body process food), higher in fiber and lower in saturated fat than traditional key lime pie.

Nutrition rundown

Carbs	Fat	Sugar	ALA	Calcium	Folic Acid
53 g	24 g	39 g	69 mg	94 mg	56 mcg

Iron	Protein	Cal	Salt	Fiber
2 mg	7 g	419	159 mg	9 g

Whole grain desert crepes with yogurt-fig-honey filling

Crepe ingredients

1 1/2 cups buckwheat flour

1/2 cup soy flour

1 1/4 cup organic low-fat milk or unsweetened soymilk

1 1/4 cup filtered water

1/2 tsp salt

Optional: 1 tsp date sugar

Cooking spray

Filling ingredients

1/2 cup figs, finely diced

1/2 cup organic unsweetened yogurt or soy yogurt

6 Tbsp honey

To make the crepe batter

Place both types of flour in a flour sifter and sift into a medium-sized mixing bowl. Add salt and mix. Place milk, date sugar, and water in a small bowl and mix well. Stir wet ingredients into the flour in 3 batches, stirring until smooth. Cover the bowl with a cloth napkin and refrigerate for one hour or overnight.

To make the dessert and dinner crepe batters together

This crepe batter is the same as that in the recipe for whole grain dinner crepes except for the addition of date sugar. If you want to make both types of crepes and are cooking for up to 3 people, divide one batch of batter in half. Use half for the dinner crepes, then add date sugar to the other half of the batter and use it for the dessert crepes. Or, to cook for 6 people, double the recipe for the dinner crepes. Then divide the batter in half and add the date sugar to one half to make the dessert batter.

To make the crepes

When batter has been cooled, remove from the refrigerator and place next to your pan. Place a cast-iron or stainless steel pan on high heat. Spray with cooking oil spray. Heat for 2 minutes. Lower heat to medium. Using a soup ladle, scoop approximately 3/4 cup of batter and pour into the middle of the pan. Place the bottom of the ladle gently on top of batter and spread batter in a circular motion. Cook for 1–2 minutes, until edges are firm and bubbles are popped. Using a spatula, gently flip crepe over. Cook the second side for 2 minutes, then remove and place on a cookie sheet.

These crepes can be made in advance and even kept overnight for easy preparation after dinner when hosting a party. If you prepared the crepes in advance, reheat them in an oven at 300 degrees for 5 minutes. Then, lay each crepe flat on a plate with the bottom (rough side) facing up. Spread 1 tablespoon of yogurt across half of the crepe, drizzle 1 teaspoon of honey and sprinkle figs on top. Fold the side without filling across the top. Makes 6 servings.

THE TASTE TEST

This nutty, wholesome take on a crepe is the closest thing you'll get to the real thing during your pregnancy without the empty carbs. Traditional crepes, made with

Radha McLean

whole eggs, butter and white (refined wheat) flour and
sold by street vendors in France, are far from nutritious.
Yet, you might imagine yourself strolling down a Parisian
lane inhaling one as you gobble up the homemade
version designed just for a woman who's pregnant. The
buckwheat and soy flour, much higher in protein, fiber,
iron and folic acid than white flour, add a nutty, hearty
flavor that's equally flavorful and much more filling
(you'll be done eating for the day after having one of
these). Plus, the yogurt-fig-honey filling is a healthy take
on a traditional dessert crepe of chocolate and bananas.

LITTLE LESSONS

Figs are a good choice of dried fruit during pregnancy
because they're high in calcium and fiber.

Honey is not only a completely natural, chemical-free
sweetener, it is known to fight toxic free radicals in the
body and has been used as a natural form of medicine for
centuries.

Nutrition rundown

Carbs	Fat	Sugar	ALA	Calcium	Folic Acid
54 g	2 g	29 g	56 mg	145 mg	50 mcg
Iron	Protein	Cal	Salt	Fiber	
2 mg	10 g	259	237 mg	5 g	

LAYERED BLONDE SPICE CAKE

This spiced twist on a traditional white cake is adapted from the multigrain coffee "cake" recipe. This version is sweeter and includes frosting, but remains deceptively lower in sugar and higher in ALA, calcium and protein than traditional cake.

Cake ingredients

2 cups soy flour

1 cup whole wheat flour

1 cup white flour

1 cup organic low-fat milk or unsweetened soymilk

1/2 cup unsweetened organic low-fat yogurt or soy yogurt

1/2 cup plus 2 tsp canola oil

1 1/2 cups maple syrup

2 Tbsp white vinegar

2 Tbsp baking powder

1 Tbsp pure vanilla extract

1 Tbsp cinnamon

1/2 tsp baking soda

1/2 tsp nutmeg

Cooking spray

Parchment paper

Optional: 1/2 cup walnuts, chopped
          1 tsp cinnamon

Frosting ingredients

1 8-ounce box organic low-fat cream cheese or vegan
    cream cheese

1/2 cup date sugar

1 Tbsp all-fruit jam

Preheat oven to 350 degrees F. Line two 9 x 9 baking
pans with parchment paper, oil each one with 1 teaspoon
canola oil, then set pans aside.

To make the cake

Place soy, whole wheat and white flours together in a
flour sifter. Sift into a mixing bowl. Place baking powder
and soda into the sifter. Sift into the bowl. Add cinnamon
and nutmeg. Stir. In a separate bowl, combine, milk,
oil, yogurt, maple syrup, vanilla, and vinegar. Stir. In 3
batches, mix wet ingredients into dry ingredients. Pour
batter, divided evenly, into prepared baking pans. Place
in oven and bake for approximately 25 minutes, until
the cakes are firm in the middle and do not stick to a
toothpick. Cool on cooling rack or cookie sheet. Remove
parchment paper from bottom of cakes.

To make the frosting

Combine cream cheese and date sugar in a bowl. Mix
with a beater or by hand until creamy. Place one cake
on a 9 x 9 cake stand. If you do not have a cake stand,
place on a cooling sheet or plate. Cover top of cake with
a thin layer of your favorite all-fruit jam. Place second
cake on top of bottom cake. Using a frosting or butter
knife, spread frosting in a thin layer evenly across top
and sides of cake, turning the cake stand, cooling sheet
or plate. Sprinkle top with chopped walnuts and/or dust

with cinnamon using a flour sifter for added color and texture. Makes 12 servings.

The taste test

This stunning blond-colored, double-layered cake is a scrumptious crowd pleaser that can be served to guests for any occasion. You will surely wow your friends and family with a dessert that looks as if you ordered it from a professional chef. Mostly importantly, though, you can *dig in* and eat a slice for dessert knowing that you're getting more vitamins and minerals from the whole wheat and soy flours than you would from only white (refined wheat) flour, which is traditionally used in baking.

Little lessons

Replacing refined wheat flour in any baking recipe with whole grain flour lowers the carb count and increases the amount of calcium, folic acid, fiber, protein, and iron.

Neither of the sugars used in this recipe is "sugar"—that is, white (refined cane) sugar—at all. Date sugar is made of ground dates, and maple syrup is a liquid taken from the maple tree. Both maple syrup and date sugar are unrefined, so they have been processed in ways that do not remove their nutrients (they both contain calcium, and date sugar even has some folic acid). They also have lower Glycemic Indexes, so they covert to less sugar in the body than white sugar—but taste just as good! Using unrefined sweeteners in baking is one way to make healthier treats for yourself and your baby.

IF YOU LIKE

If you like nuts, then add them! Chopped walnuts would add ALA, calcium, and zinc. You can add them to the batter, sprinkle them on top of the cake, or both.

LITTLE TIPS

You can make the flour mixture in advance, or double the recipe and store it in the freezer for up to 3 months.

For a wheat-free recipe, use barley or spelt flour instead of wheat flour. For a gluten-free recipe, use gluten-free baking mix instead of whole wheat flour.

Nutrition rundown

Carbs	Fat	Sugar	ALA	Calcium	Folic Acid
58 g	18 g	32 g	2 g	308 mg	65 mcg

Iron	Protein	Cal	Salt	Fiber
3 mg	10 g	420	396 mg	4 g

PROTEIN DREAM CHOCOLATE PUDDING

1 15-ounce block silken (soft) tofu

3 Tbsp maple syrup

1 12-ounce bag grain-sweetened chocolate chips*

Place chocolate chips in a stainless steel bowl. Fill a double boiler halfway with water and bring water to a boil. Place bowl with chips on top of the boiler. With a whisk or mixing spoon, stir the chips continually until they are melted. Immediately turn off the heat. Or, place the chips in a ceramic bowl and heat in the microwave on high for 15—30 seconds. The chips should be almost completely melted.

Crumble the block of tofu and place it in a blender. Add the maple syrup and melted chocolate. Cover and puree for 30 seconds to 1 minute, until smooth.

Spoon pudding into 4 individual dessert cups. Place cups on a tray, over with cloth napkin and place in refrigerator. Refrigerate for at least 1 hour, but ideally for 3 hours or more. Serve chilled and eat quickly! For added color, sprinkle fresh berries a chiffonade of mint leaves (by stacking the leaves, rolling them tightly, then cutting across the rolled leaves with a sharp knife, producing fine ribbons) on top. Makes 4 servings.

THE TASTE TEST

You won't believe your taste buds when you swallow this sensuously creamy and divinely rich dessert. The beauty of how delicious it is lies in the fact that it's so easy to make, lower in fat and higher in protein and nutrients

Radha McLean

relative to traditional pudding made with white (refined cane) sugar, heavy cream, and eggs.

LITTLE LESSONS

Silken tofu is a *pièce de résistance* (special item) in the kitchen for dessert lovers who want alternatives to cooking with heavy cream and eggs. Its smooth consistency and inherent ability to firm up when refrigerated makes it an ingenious ingredient for quiches and puddings.

Grain-sweetened chocolate ships are healthier for you because they're sweetened with grains instead of white sugar.

*One brand of grain-sweetened chocolate ships is Sunspire. Contact information for Sunspire can be found in the Resources chapter.

Nutrition rundown

Carbs	Fat	Sugar	ALA	Calcium	Folic Acid
53 g	22 g	28 g	285 mg	139	51 mcg
Iron	Protein	Cal	Salt	Fiber	
2	12	425	11	5	

Resources

CLEANING SUPPLIES

Homemade cleaning supplies

Earth Easy
www.eartheasy.com/live_nontoxic_solutions.htm

Pioneer Thinking
www.pioneerthinking.com/homecleaning1.html

About My Planet
www.aboutmyplanet.com/daily-green-tips/cleaning-products

Information on toxins

Environmental Protection Agency, Inside the Home
www.epa.gov/iaq/voc.html

COMPOSTING

How to Compost
www.howtocompost.org

FISH ADVISORIES

Environmental Protection Agency local fish advisory
www.epa.gov/waterscience/fish/states.htm

Natural Resources Defense Council mercury guide
www.nrdc.org/health/effects/mercury/guide.asp

FOOD

Brands listed in recipes

Ancient Harvest
http://www.quinoa.net

Arrowhead Mills
www.arrowheadmills.com

Barbara's Bakery
www.barbarasbakery.com

Bragg Liquid Aminos
http://bragg.com/products/la.html

Custom Chocolate Shop
www.customchocolateshop.com

Good Morning
www.goodmorningcereals.com

House Foods Tofu Shirataki noodles
www.house-foods.com/tofushirataki_faq.html

I.M. Healthy
www.soynutbutter.com

Nature's Path
www.naturespath.com

Pero
www.internaturalfoods.com/Pero/Pero.html

Red Star nutritional yeast flakes
www.redstaryeast.com

Sunspire
www.sunspire.com

Carbonated drinks, all-natural

Crystal Geyser
www.crystalgeyserasw.com

Izze
www.izze.com

RW Knudsen
www.knudsenjuices.com

Farmers Markets

Local Harvest
www.localharvest.org

Organic Consumers Association
www.organicconsumers.org

Nutrition during pregnancy

United States Department of Agriculture (USDA)
MyPyramid
www.mypyramid.gov/mypyramidmoms/index.html

Dolan, Deirdre and Alexandra Zissu. *The Complete Organic Pregnancy*. New York: Harper Collins, 2006.

Omega-3 Fat

Deva Nutrition algae-based DHA supplement
www.devanutrition.com/vegan_DHA.html

Tribole, Evelyn, RD. *The Ultimate Omega-3 Diet*. New York: McGraw-Hill, 2007.

Organic food

Diamond Organics
www.diamondorganics.com

Fresh Direct
www.freshdirect.com/index.jsp

Door to Door Organics
www.doortodoororganics.com

Organic Direct
www.organicdirect.com

Organic Consumers Association
www.organicconsumers.org

Green Restaurant Association
www.dinegreen.com

Trader Joe's
www.traderjoes.com

Whole Foods Market
www.wholefoodsmarket.com

Food Safety

Centers for Disease Control and Prevention
Listeriosis
www.cdc.gov/nczved/dfbmd/disease_listing/listeriosis_gi.html

GREEN LIVING

Environmental Working Group
www.ewg.org

Smith, Alicia Marie. *50 Plus One Tips for Going Green.* Chicago: Encouragement Press, 2007.

The Green Network, cable television (check local listings for channel in your area)

Tree Hugger
www.treehugger.com

HEALTHCARE PROVIDERS

American Association of Naturopathic Physicians
http://www.naturopathic.org

American Dietetic Association
www.eatright.org

RECYCLING

National Recycling Coalition
www.nrc-recycle.org

McCorquodale, Duncan and Cigalle Hanaor. *Recycle: The Essential Guide.* London: Black Dog Publishing, 2006.

RICE COOKER, ALUMINUM-FREE

The New Miracle Rice Cooker
www.miracleexclusives.net

WATER FILTERS

Aquasana
www.aquasana.com

Multi-Pure Drinking Water Systems
www.multipureco.com

Ionized/alkaline water–AKAI filter
www.hightechhealth.com

Kangen Water USA
www.kangenwaterusa.com

All Internet links were active at time of publication.

Notes

1. United States Department of Agriculture Organic Production/Organic Food, "What is organic production?" www.nal.usda.gov/afsic/pubs/ofp/ofp. shtml.

2. RW Clapp et al., "Environmental and Occupational Causes of Cancer: New Evidence 2005–2007," *Rev Environ Health* 23 (2008): 1–37.

3. F Xue F et al., "Maternal Fish Consumption, Mercury Levels, and Risk of Preterm Delivery," *Environ Health Perspect* 115 (2007): 42–47.

4. AS Holmes et al., "Reduced Levels of Mercury in First Baby Haircuts of Autistic Children," *Int J Toxicol* 22 (2003): 277–285.

5. E Oken et al., "Maternal Fish Intake During Pregnancy, Blood Mercury Levels, and Child Cognition at Age 3 Years in a US Cohort," *Am J Epidemiol* 167 (2008): 1171–1181.

6. Joanna Burger et al., "Mercury in Commercial Fish: Optimizing Individual Choices to Reduce Risk," *Environmental Health Perspectives* 113 (2005): 266–271.

7. Natural Resources Defense Council, "Consumer Guide to Mercury in Fish," www.nrdc.org/health/effects/mercury/guide.asp.

8. U.S. Environmental Protection Agency, "Fish Advisories," www.epa.gov/waterscience/fish/states. htm.

9. Jeanne-Marie Bartas, "Aquaculture: An Overview," *Vegetarian Journal,* May/June 1997.

10. CJ Creighton et al., "Insulin-like Growth Factor-I

Activates Gene Transcription Programs Strongly Associated with Poor Breast Cancer Prognosis," *J Clin Oncol 26 (2008): 4060–4062.*

11. Food and Agriculture Organization of the United Nations, *Livestock's Long Shadow. Environmental Issues and Options,* 2006.

12. Environmental Defense Fund, "Fighting Global Warming with Food: Low-Carbon Choices for Dinner," www.edf.org/article.cfm?contentid=6604.

13. Mark Bittman, "Putting Meat Back in Its Place," *The New York Times*, June 11, 2008, Dining and Wine section.

14. Institute of Medicine, "Dietary Reference Intakes: Macronutrients," September 2002, www.iom.edu/Object.File/Master/7/300/Webtablemacro.pdf.

15. American Dietetic Association, "Position of the American Dietetic Association: Nutrition and Lifestyle for a Healthy Pregnancy Outcome," *Journal of the American Dietetic Association* 102 (2002): 1479–1490.

16. United States Department of Agriculture, "MyPyramid for Pregnancy and Breastfeeding," www.mypyramid.gov/mypyramidmoms/index.html.

17. Institute of Medicine. *Dietary Reference Intakes for Calcium, Phosphate, Magnesium, Vitamin D, and Fluoride* (Washington, DC: National Academy Press, 1997).

18. American Dietetic Association, "Position of the American Dietetic Association and Dietitians of Canada: Vegetarian Diets," *American Dietetic Association Reports* 106 (2003) doi: 10.1053/jada.2003.50142.

19. United States Department of Agriculture National

Nutrient Database for Standard Reference, Release 20, "Nutrient Lists," Sept, 26, 2007, www.ars.usda.gov/Main/docs.htm?docid=15869.

20. Centers for Disease Control and Prevention, "Recommendations to Prevent and Control Iron Deficiency in the United States," *MMWR* 47 (1998): 1–36.

21. Institute of Medicine, "Dietary Reference Intakes for Energy, Carbohydrate, Fiber, Fat, Fatty Acids, Cholesterol, Protein, and Amino Acids," September 2002, www.iom.edu/CMS/3788/4576/4340.aspx.

22. B Koletzko et al., "Dietary Fat Intake for Pregnant and Lactating Women," *British J Nutr* (2007): 1–5.

23. E Oken et al., "Maternal Fish Intake During Pregnancy, Blood Mercury Levels, and Child Cognition at Age 3 Years in a US Cohort," *Am J Epidemiol* 167 (2008): 1171–1181.

24. TA Sanders, "Essential Fatty Acid Requirements of Vegetarians in Pregnancy, Lactation, and Infancy," *Am J Clin Nutr* 70(3 Suppl), 1999: 555S–559S.

25. Paula Kurtzweil, "Daily Values Encourage Healthy Diet," *Food and Drug Administration Special Issue Consumer,* May 1993, http://www.fda.gov/fdac/foodlabel/special.html

26. Centers for Disease Control and Prevention, "Listeriosis," www.cdc.gov/nczved/dfbmd/disease_listing/listeriosis_gi.html.

27. Anne Christiansen Bullers, "Bottled Water: Better Than the Tap?" *FDA Consumer* magazine, July–August 2002. www.fda.gov/FDAC/features/2002/402_h2o.html.

ABOUT THE AUTHOR AND CONTRIBUTORS

Radha McLean is a journalist specializing in health and medicine who has been published in numerous magazines including *Diabetes Health, Nurseweek,* and *Pregnancy.* She is a lifelong vegetarian who grew up cooking and eating organic food. Ms. McLean, 37, now lives a green lifestyle with her husband and 2-year-old son in New York City.

Tara Gidus, MS, RD, CSSD, LD/N, is a nationally-recognized expert on nutrition, fitness and health promotion. As a National Media Spokesperson for the American Dietetic Association, Tara is quoted in a variety of media, including television, newspapers, magazines and Web sites. Most importantly, she is the mother of one boy, Basil.

Dr. Thauna Abrin, ND, is a Defeat Autism Now and midwifery-trained naturopathic doctor in private practice in the San Francisco Bay Area. Dr. Abrin passionately believes that following both a healthy diet and preconception detoxification helps to ensure a healthy pregnancy and baby. She can be reached at www. drthauna.com.